ZANG FU 臟腑
The Organ Systems of Traditional Chinese Medicine

ZANG FU 臟腑

The Organ Systems of Traditional Chinese Medicine

Functions, Interrelationships and Patterns of Disharmony in Theory and Practice

Jeremy Ross

Doctor of Acupuncture
CAc(Nanjing) BAc(MBAcA) BSc CEd MNIMH

Second Edition

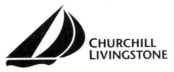

CHURCHILL
LIVINGSTONE

EDINBURGH LONDON MADRID MELBOURNE AND NEW YORK 1985

CHURCHILL LIVINGSTONE
An imprint of Harcourt Brace and Company Limited

© Jeremy Ross 1994
© Longman Group Limited 1985
© Pearson Professional Limited 1998
© Harcourt Brace and Company Limited 1998

🖉 is a registered trademark of Harcourt Brace and
Company Limited

First edition 1984
Second edition 1985
    Reprinted 1986
    Reprinted 1987
    Reprinted 1988
    Reprinted 1989
    Reprinted 1990
    Reprinted 1993
    Reprinted 1994
    Reprinted 1995
    Reprinted 1998 (twice)

ISBN 0-443-03482-6

British Library Cataloguing in Publication Data
A catalogue record for this book is available from the
British Library

**Library of Congress Cataloging in Publication
Data**
A catalog record for this book is available from the
Library of Congress

Printed in Hong Kong
WC/11

The
publisher's
policy is to use
**paper manufactured
from sustainable forests**

Preface
to the Second Edition

In this new edition, certain sections have been extensively revised, and much new material has been added. In the first edition, students found **Part I The Background** especially helpful in understanding Zang Fu, and in seeing the organ systems in the context of Chinese Thought and Chinese Physiology. In response to their requests and their enthusiasm, the sections on Origins and Patterns of Disease have been greatly expanded with many new Tables and Figures.

Also, since the emphasis of this book is on the practical applications of Zang Fu theory, two more Case Histories have been added to Chapter 18. In addition, various minor alterations and corrections have been made to the text.

Bristol 1985   Jeremy Ross

Acknowledgements

To the staff of Nanjing College of TCM, and of Zhongsan Medical College, without whom this book would not have been possible.

In particular, to my tutor Dr Su Xin Ming for his patience and thorough explanations, and to Professor Wu Xinjin.

To Sheila Roberts for her help with editing and word processing.

J.R.

Dedicated to my Father with Love and Respect

Contents

Introduction

The practice of Traditional Chinese Acupuncture is largely based on a framework of three interwoven categories:

Jing Luo
Eight Principles
Zang Fu

The Eight Principles have been clearly dealt with in recent texts, and their fundamental importance is now beginning to be understood.

The importance of Jing Luo, the system of channels and collaterals, is one of the few things that has been appreciated in Western Acupuncture from its beginnings.

The theory of Zang Fu forms the core of Traditional Chinese Medicine (TCM) and yet has received the least attention and has been subject to the grossest misconceptions.

This text deals with the Zang Fu, their functions, Origins of Disease, and Patterns of Disharmony. It studies their interrelationships with each other, with the Substances, Jing Luo, and Tissues, and with the Origins of Disease. It views them in the context of the Body as a whole, in its interactions with the environment.

The Purpose of This Book

This book aims to:

1. Provide a clear, well organized foundation for a theoretical understanding of Zang Fu.
2. Explore the interwoven complexities of Zang Fu interrelationships, and to clarify areas of difficulty and ambiguity.

3. Show how Zang Fu theory is applied in practice, and to provide a basic sequence of clinical procedures.

This book is an advanced acupuncture text. It is written for students and practitioners of TCM, and is not meant for the complete beginner. It assumes some degree of familiarity with the theory and practice of TCM, and is meant to be used in conjunction with such excellent texts as 'Essentials of Chinese Acupuncture' (9), 'Acupuncture A Comprehensive Text' (18), and 'The Web That Has No Weaver' (12).

It is concerned with one main topic, the application of the Theory of Zang Fu in clinical practice. It deals with other topics, for example, Substances, only in sufficient detail to give an adequate background to the Theory of Zang Fu, and assumes that the reader either has knowledge of these other topics or has access to the textbooks mentioned above.

How This Book is Organized

The main body of this book is divided into four parts:

Part 1 The Background
Part 2 Zang Fu
Part 3 Interrelationships
Part 4 Clinical Practice

The whole purpose of this book would be defeated if the reader were to omit Part 1, and go straight to Part 2. The Zang Fu can only really be understood in the context of the basic principles of TCM.

Part 1
This section looks at the fundamental differences between Chinese and Western thought, and at the main theoretical principles of Chinese medicine. It considers Zang Fu in the context of the basic organizational framework of the Body: Substances, Jing Luo and Tissues; and in terms of the Origins of Disease.

Part 2
This part is of course the core of the book, but meaningless out of the context of Part 1 and Part 3.

After a general introduction to Zang Fu, Part 2 discusses each Zang Fu pair in a separate chapter; and studies the functions, Origins of Disease, and Patterns of Disharmony of each Zang in detail, with many examples, tables and diagrams.

Part 3
Interrelationship is the basic theme of this book, and this vital section explores the interrelationships of Zang Fu with Yin Yang, Jing Luo, Tissues, emotions and behaviour, and Origins of Disease. It investigates the interrelationships between Zang Fu in disharmonies involving two, three or more Zang Fu together.

Part 4

Deals with the treatment of Zang Fu disharmonies in clinical practice, and discusses details of diagnosis, treatment, and the education of the patient. It considers analysis of pulse and tongue, choice and use of points, and gives a simple sequence of procedures for clinical practice. Finally, there are detailed analyses of selected case histories.

Theory and Practice

The emphasis of this book is on the practical application of theoretical principles in the clinic, not upon theory for its own sake. In TCM, theory and practice are mutually dependent, each refines and advances the other.

If theory is not consistently confirmed by clinical experience, then it must be discarded or refined. It is the theory that must be altered to match the facts; the facts must never be twisted to match the theory.

Figures

In the Figures in this book, lines with an arrow, →, represent a movement mainly in one direction, whereas lines without an arrow, ——, signify that movement can be in either direction. For example:

Deficient Shen Yang → Deficient Pi Yang

indicates that Deficient Shen Yang tends to give rise to Deficient Pi Yang, rather than vice versa. In contrast to this:

Blazing Gan Fire —— Damp Heat in Gan and Dan

Indicates that either Blazing Gan Fire may give rise to Damp heat in Gan and Dan, or vice versa, depending on the circumstances, and that movement is not predominantly in one direction.

Useful Lists

Warning

Acupuncture points mentioned in this book are **NOT** meant to be used as symptomatic prescriptions. Point selection must always be for a specific individual, under particular circumstances at a particular time; and must be based on a thorough understanding of the origins of the Pattern of Disharmony of that individual.

List of Chinese Words

The use of Chinese words has been kept to a minimum, but where a concept in TCM has no accurate English equivalent, the Chinese word is used throughout:

General

Zang Fu	The organ systems of TCM
Zang	The Yin organ systems
Fu	The Yang organ systems
Jing Luo	The system of channels and collaterals
Xue Mai	The system of channels and collaterals carrying predominantly Xue
Ming Men	Gate of Life

Substances

Chinese words	English approximation
Qi	Energy
Xue	Blood
Jing	Essence
Shen*	Spirit
Jin Ye	Body Fluids

Types of Qi

Chinese words	English approximation
Yuan Qi	Original Qi
Gu Qi	Grain Qi
Zong Qi	Qi of Chest
Zhen Qi	True Qi
Ying Qi	Nutritive Qi
Wei Qi	Defensive Qi

Zang Fu

Zang

Chinese words	English approximation	Abbreviation
Shen	Kidneys	KID
Pi	Spleen	SP
Gan	Liver	LIV
Xin	Heart	HE
Fei	Lungs	LU
Xin Bao	Pericardium	P

Fu

Chinese words	English approximation	Abbreviation
Pang Guang	Bladder	BL
Wei	Stomach	ST
Dan	Gall Bladder	GB
Xiao Chang	Small Intestine	SI
Da Chang	Large Intestine	LI
San Jiao	Triple Burner	TB

Eight Miscellaneous Channels
(Eight Extra Meridians)

Chinese words	English Approximation	Chinese words	English Approximation
Du Mai	Governing Channel	Yang Qiao Mai	Yang Heel Channel
Ren Mai	Conception Channel	Yin Qiao Mai	Yin Heel Channel
Chong Mai	Penetrating Channel	Yin Wei Mai	Yin Linking Channel
Dai Mai	Girdle Channel	Yang Wei Mai	Yang Linking Channel

Conventions

Generally speaking, each Chinese concept is represented by a single Chinese character, or by a group of two or more characters. Chinese characters are not used in this book, and the convention adopted is that when a Chinese concept is composed of more than one character, each character is represented by a single Chinese word in Western script, beginning with a capital letter. For example, the term Jing Luo represents a group of two characters, and the term Bu Nei Wai Yin represents a group of four characters.

This convention is arbitrary, and various representations are found in other texts, for example, Jing Luo, Jing-luo, Jingluo, jing luo, jing-luo, and jingluo.

The exception to this convention is the Chinese names of the acupuncture points, which have been written as single words even when deriving from two or more characters, since this is the convention adopted by many other tests. For example, Du 4 is written as Mingmen, not as Ming Men.

The Pinyin system of spelling has been used throughout; and the system of names and numbers for the so-called 'New' and 'Miscellaneous' acupuncture points is that used in 'Acupuncture, a Comprehensive Text' (18). There are rare exceptions, eg. there is no apparent equivalent in (18) for Chuanhsi, which is listed in (1) and (10). Chuanhsi is therefore written in the Wade-Giles notation, and without a number.

To keep the use of Chinese words to a minimum, certain English words and phrases are used as translations or approximations of Chinese words. For example the Chinese word Xu is translated by the English word Deficiency. Such English words begin with capitals to emphasize that they stand for a Chinese concept.

Book titles have been put in inverted commas, for example, 'I Jing', 'Nei Jing', and 'Essentials of Chinese Acupuncture'.

Part

1

The Background

Chapter

1

Chinese and Western Thought

The greatest difficulty for the Western student of Traditional Chinese Medicine (TCM) lies in the tremendous differences between Western and Chinese patterns of thought.

Few Western practitioners are aware of the full extent of these differences, and few are prepared to spend time and energy in understanding them. Many practitioners adopt a Western mental approach in dealing with Chinese concepts, or even attempt to force Western concepts into the Chinese system. The resulting mish-mash is, by definition, no longer TCM.

The more practitioners can leave aside Western pre-conceptions and styles of thinking, the more they can adopt a Chinese mental approach. This will lead them to a fuller understanding of TCM, and to improved results in clinical practice.

Patterns of Change

The Chinese view the Universe as an infinite network of interweaving energy flows; the transient nodes in this ever-changing network representing events in space and time.

They view all areas of the network as inter-communicating and inter-dependent; any given area only having existence and meaning within the context of the whole. The principle of interrelationship is constant, but the patterns of relationship are ever-changing; the network is in constant movement and transformation.

Within this vast network, this greater pattern, it is possible for man to perceive subsidiary patterns, indeed the entire Universe can be represented by the 64 Hexagrams or Transformations of the 'I Jing' (11). If these basic patterns are thoroughly understood, it is possible to perceive the pattern underlying a particular time and situation, to project back into the past, to show the origins of the pattern; and forward into the future to predict its development. With this understanding, the action appropriate to a particular time and situation can be performed.

This has obvious application to medical practice with respect to diagnosis, treatment, prognosis and the education of the patient. Understanding of the pattern of particular patients, in the context of their environment at a particular time, gives understanding of their past history and of their future. This is not simply a matter of mysticism, but of standard clinical practice.

In Western conception, the word 'pattern' tends to indicate a fixed static structure, like a blue-print or a mould, contrasting with the Chinese conception of an association of functional relationships. Throughout this book, the word pattern is used in the Chinese conception.

Emphasis is above all on movement, not upon set structures existing at a set time, but upon transformations. The structures temporarily generated by the changes are of secondary interest to the changes themselves.

Interrelationship

Interrelationship is a recurring theme throughout this book. Nothing exists in isolation.

In general terms, it is the interrelationship between the different phenomena within a pattern which is important, and the interrelationship of the different patterns to each other within the context of the whole.

In human terms, all depends upon the interrelationship of the different patterns within an individual, and of that individual to others and to the natural environment.

In terms of the Zang Fu, the interactions of the individual with the environment reflect the interrelationships of the Zang Fu with each other, and with the Substances, Jing Luo, and Tissues, within the framework of the Body as a whole.

Analysis and Synthesis

Generally, with some notable exceptions, for example modern physics and ecology, Western thinking does not tend to look for overall patterns, nor does it tend to look at the whole or at the parts in the context of the whole. Western thought still tends to view events or individuals as discreet particles, very like the balls on a billiard table, interacting only when they collide, and not having any interpenetration or intercommunication with each other. Therefore, it is seen as easy and permissible to study one of these particles in isolation from its environment. Generally, Western research tries to minimise the number of variables and reduces the phenomenon to its simplest elements, so that each can be studied separately.

In relative terms, Western thinking tends to be reductive and analytic, whereas Chinese thinking tends to be synthetic and intuitive. Where the Chinese attempt synthesis, by arranging different phenomena into patterns, at its most simplistic,

Western science attempts to reduce phenomena to their simplest possible components, and to relate the different components to each other in linear chains of cause and effect:-

$$A \rightarrow B \rightarrow C \rightarrow D \rightarrow$$
$$\downarrow \qquad\qquad \text{etc.}$$
$$E \rightarrow F \rightarrow$$

A corollary of this lies in attitudes to time. The Western approach arranges events in a linear time sequence, whereas the Chinese think in terms of the synchronous occurrence of the different phenomena that form a particular pattern.

This extreme form of Western thought arose from the same background of Western philosophy and culture that gave rise to Classical Physics, specifically, Newtonian Mechanics, the physics of separate particles.

In complete contrast to this, the concepts of modern physics give a picture increasingly similar to the Chinese world view (4). However, current medicine and technology are still deeply imbued with the old ideas of separate particles and fixed structures, and the concepts of modern physics may take years to filter through to the medical sciences and to Western culture.

This problem was aggravated by the mechanisation and urbanisation consequent upon the Industrial Revolution. This involved a movement away from the patterns of the countryside and the natural world, and an increasing tendency to view man and other living organisms in terms of machines.

In its worst aspects, this is associated with the tendency in general theory to separate part from part, and the part from the whole; with the great problems of the modern world associated with the separation of man from his inner self, from his fellow men, and from nature; and with the tendency of medical practice to separate the patient from the disease, and from the environment.

This approach to medicine tends to view the body as a machine and to treat it accordingly. It sees disease as an external thing that the patient 'catches by chance', separable from the patient by treatment.

Where the Chinese synthesise as complete a pattern as possible, Western medicine tends to isolate a single causative factor, i.e. to reduce the situation to its simplest possible component. An inevitable corollary to this, is that whilst TCM treats the individual as a whole, Western medicine tends to treat the disease and not the patient.

Yin Yang

The concept of Yin Yang forms a recurring theme throughout this book and it is the basis of Chinese medicine.

The Western tendency is to view opposites as absolutes; the words black and white give this impression. This derives from the tendency to see the world as made up of discreet particles, and from a desire to be as precise as possible. Hence a situation is either:-

a or **b**

The Chinese view such phenomena as the two extremes of a continuum:-

or, more precisely:-

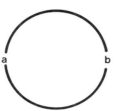

These terms are relative; not black and white, but blacker and whiter. Also, the polarity is never static; it is in continual change, blacker becoming whiter and vice versa. This idea has important ramifications.

Energy and Matter
In TCM, energy and matter are not seen as separate, but as the two extremes of a continuum. For example, Westerners tend to view Qi as energy, and Xue (Blood) as matter. The Chinese view it differently; there are denser, more material aspects of Qi just as there are lighter, more energetic aspects of Xue. In this book, the word Substances is used to include Qi, Xue, Jing (Essence), Shen* (Spirit), and Jin Ye (Body Fluids); without implications of the relative proportions of energy or matter, Yin or Yang.

Mind and Body
Western thinking similarly tends to separate mind from body, and spiritual from material. In TCM, each of the pairs, mind and body, and spirit and matter, is regarded as a continuum.

Structure and Function

Structure and function represent a further Western dichotomy; structure being the material framework and function being the results of a flow of energy through that framework. Chinese thought sees structure and function as a continuum, and does not distinguish between them. They are not viewed as separate areas, and separate textbooks of anatomy and physiology are not a feature of Traditional Chinese Medicine.

Western medicine tends to see everything in terms of structure, from morphology and anatomy down through histology to molecular biochemistry. Function is seen in terms of structure, as is pathology, and diseases tend to refer to structures. Chinese medicine is completely different; it emphasizes function. Little emphasis is placed on structure, especially internal structures. Hence the Zang Fu, the organ systems of TCM, do not refer so much to structures as to functions.

Precision and Ambiguity

Generally, in dealing with words, concepts and definitions, Western science aims for precision, involving reduction to the smallest, clearest element. Chinese concepts, however, like Chinese characters or the Hexagrams of the 'I Jing', are situational:- the meaning depends not just on the word itself, but also on the context, the particular situation of time and place. Chinese concepts also interweave and overlap so that to a Westerner, they may appear vague, imprecise, ambiguous, confusing and blurred. They are flexible, open to different interpretations, with various shades of meaning, depending upon the context. Where the Westerner tries to restrict the meaning, Chinese thought tends to open it up so that it can be linked with as many other patterns are possible.

In TCM, this leads to difficulties in translation, especially of the ancient texts, to the confusion and irritation of Western students. It also leads to gross misunderstanding, and to innumerable attempts to force Chinese concepts into Western moulds, and vice versa.

Harmony and Disharmony

Western Medicine reflects Western thinking in Western Society, tending to an aggressive, combative approach in which the disease area is cut, burnt, irradiated, injected or subjected to other suppressive chemical treatment. Chinese medicine is completely different. The ultimate aim of Chinese philosophy and culture is harmony. Harmony within an individual, within the family, within the state, and between man and the natural world. By recognising the patterns within nature, and by acting in harmony with them, man not only preserves his health but fulfils himself.

The practitioner of TCM is not trying to isolate a disease agent and wage war against it, but to perceive a pattern of disharmony and to treat it in such a way as to help the Body itself to restore harmony.

Summary

It must be remembered that by contrasting Western and Chinese thought in this rather drastic manner, we are only emphasizing the extremes of a continuum. Both modes of thought contain elements of each other, and this is especially so today since there has been much recent interchange between the two cultures.

Each system has its strengths and weaknesses, and each has developed a particular area of human understanding. The two systems are complimentary. However, whereas TCM is basically a complete and finished system based on ancient texts and their commentaries, modern Western medicine is, relatively, in its infancy.

Eventually, as true TCM becomes more thoroughly understood and more accurately applied in the West, and as Western medicine grows and matures over the years, an evolving systhesis will develop both in theory and in practice; but the time for this is not yet. Premature attempts to mix Chinese and Western concepts only lead to confusion, and, in the West, to poor understanding and practice of TCM.

Chapter
2

The Framework

In the West, the word 'body' indicates the physical aspect; 'the body' as distinct from 'the mind', or 'the body' as distinct from 'the spirit'. In this book, the word 'Body' implies not only the complex of physical, emotional, mental and spiritual aspects, but also the ongoing interaction between this complex and the external environment. This interaction manifests as the changing patterns of behaviour that are variously termed the 'way of life', the 'lifestyle', or simply the 'life' of the individual.

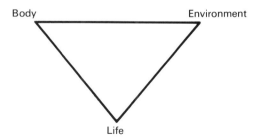

In Western medicine, the emphasis is on a structural framework; bones, muscles and other tissues, inhabited by the organs, and permeated and integrated by the blood, endocrine and nervous systems. In Chinese medicine, the emphasis is on a framework of functional interrelationships. TCM is more concerned with the functional aspects of the Zang Fu, and the Substances that flow through them, than with their structures.

In TCM, there is a functional framework of four main interwoven categories:-

Substances
Jing Luo
Zang Fu
Tissues

By the action of the Zang Fu, the basic Substances are transformed and transported, especially via Jing Luo, to all the Tissues of the Body.

Substances

The basic substances of TCM are Qi (Energy), Xue (Blood), Jing (Essence), Shen★ (Spirit) and Jin Ye (Body Fluids).

The term Substances does not imply energy or matter; all is relative.
For example, Wei Qi (Defensive Qi) is relatively more energetic, Ying Qi (Nutritive Qi) is relatively more material. Jing is relatively more material than Qi but less material than Xue.
The Substances are the subject of the next chapter.

Jing Luo

There is considerable vagueness and ambiguity surrounding the use of the terms Jing, Mai and Luo; and their combinations Jing Luo, Jing Mai and Luo Mai.

Mai
This term has two main meanings:-

The Pulse
The Vessels

Mai may indicate the pulse in the sense of the rhythmic, pulsating movement of the Substances in the vessels; and it may also indicate the vessels themselves, in terms of the network that limits and directs the movement of Qi and Xue within the Body.

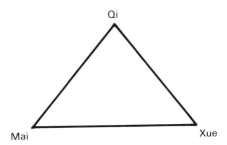

There is an interdependence of Qi, Xue and Mai, in which Qi provides the dynamic force associated with the movement of the Substances through the vessels; Xue is the more substantial aspect, filling the vessels and being confined by them;

and Mai is both the system of vessels containing the Substances, and the rhythmic pulsations in the movement of the Substances in the vessels.

Hence, it is said that 'Mai moves in accordance with Qi' and that 'Xue moves in accordance with Mai Qi'. Also, that 'Mai confines the Qi' and that 'Xue moves within the Mai'.

In common use, Mai means veins, but in Traditional medical use, Mai indicates the system of pathways through which the Substances, especially Qi and Xue, are distributed around the Body. The term Xue Mai is sometimes used to indicate that part of the Mai system more concerned with the movement of Xue, than with the movement of Qi. The Xue Mai system has superficial resemblances to the vascular system of Western medicine, but there are fundamental differences.

Mai is therefore a term which includes those systems which carry predominantly Qi, and those which carry predominantly Xue; but little distinction may be made between these systems, and the exact meaning of Mai will depend on the context.

Jing

Jing refers to the warp threads in a piece of fabric, and has the meaning of 'to go through', 'to steer through', or 'to direct'. In TCM, Jing refers to the network of energy pathways. The term Jing Mai means 'to direct energy through definite pathways'. In practice, the terms Jing, Mai and Jing Mai, may be used interchangeably to refer to the system of pathways through which Qi and Xue move around the Body. The Jing Mai system is variously referred to as pathways, meridians, conduits, channels or vessels. The use of the word Jing, in this sense, may be differentiated from the word Jing meaning Essence, by the context.

Jing Luo

Jing means 'to direct', and Luo means 'a net', 'a network', 'a connecting or attaching system'. Jing or Jing Mai may refer to the main vessels or channels; and Luo or Luo Mai may refer to the branch vessels or collaterals. Hence, Jing Luo is often translated as 'channels and collaterals'. For example, the phrase 'Dan Jing Luo' refers to the channels and collaterals, or main and branching vessels of Dan.

There is a common misconception that Jing Luo, or Jing Mai, carry Qi, whereas Xue Mai carry Xue. Jing Luo carry both Qi and Xue, and indeed certain texts translate Jing Luo as 'blood vessels' (16).

The Jing Luo system of channels and collaterals, forms a network of pathways connecting together all parts of the Body, so that the Substances, especially Qi and Xue, may be transported between all the Zang Fu and Tissue systems. Jing Luo, though invisible, are considered to have a definate physical reality, but this reality is more in terms of functions than of structure.

Acupuncture Points

All acupuncture treatment is based upon the use of the acupuncture points. These points upon the channels, just below the surface of the body, at specific anatomical locations, represent points at which the flow of Substances within the channels can be adjusted in order to restore harmony.

The Jing Luo, their distribution and patterns of disharmony, and the acupuncture points and their indications, are dealt with thoroughly elsewhere (9 & 18), and will not be considered separately in this book.

Zang Fu

The Zang Fu may be described as the organ systems of Chinese medicine, providing it is understood that they are organ systems in terms of functional interrelationships, rather than in terms of specific structures, and that they do not correspond to the organ systems of Western medicine.

Tissues

The main tissues of TCM are the Bones, Tendons, Flesh, Blood Vessels and Skin.

The eyes, ears, nose, mouth and tongue are regarded as the upper orifices or as the sense organs, depending on the context; the lower orifices being those of the anus, urethra and genitals.

The Curious Organs are the Marrow, Brain, Bones, Uterus, Blood Vessels and Gall Bladder. Bones and Blood Vessels are regarded as Tissues or as Curious Organs, depending on the context.

The Tissues are perhaps the nearest thing to structures in Chinese medicine, but their importance must still be considered more in terms of their function, and of their interrelationships with the other systems in the Body.

Summary

There is an exchange of energy and materials between the Body and the external environment: air, food and drink entering the Body, and waste materials leaving it. The Zang Fu are involved in this interchange with the environment, and also, within the Body, in the metabolism of the basic Substances, and in their transportation, mainly via Jing Luo and Xue Mai, to all parts of the Body, including the Tissues, Orifices and Curious Organs.

Chapter

3

Substances

The Five Substances and Their Functions

The five main categories of the basic Substances of TCM, are listed in Table 3.1 with their English language approximations. The Chinese words are used in this book, since the English words give rise to many misconceptions.

Table 3.1 The Five Main Substances

Chinese words	English approximation
Qi	Energy
Xue	Blood
Jing	Essence
Shen*	Spirit
Jin Ye	Body Fluids

For example, the term Qi is used in preference to Energy, since the latter implies energy as opposed to matter. In TCM, energy-matter is a continuum, Qi having both energetic and material attributes.

Similarly, Shen* is used in preference to Spirit, since the latter implies spirit as opposed to body, or spiritual as opposed to material, and, in the context of TCM, Shen* may have material aspects.

Western words can be most misleading when applied to Chinese concepts, since the Western words do not give the sense of the Chinese ideas, but carry with them their Western meanings. For example, Xue is used rather than Blood, since the latter implies the blood of Western medicine, with its precise parameters of biochemistry and histology. Although Xue and blood share some common attributes, fundamentally, Xue is a different concept.

The basic emphasis in Western medicine is on structure, e.g. the detailed structure of the blood vessels and the detailed composition of the blood that passes through them. TCM is little concerned with structure, with the histology of the Jing Luo or the chemical composition of Qi; its concern is with their functions and with the relationships between them. Most of all, TCM is concerned with pathology. In a Chinese text there is almost no discussion of structure; there is a certain amount of physiology, but the bulk of the book is usually on the patterns of disease and their treatment.

The interwoven complexity of the functional interrelationships of the Substances, means that it is difficult to separate one from another with precise definitions. Indeed, TCM is not concerned with such precision; the meaning of words is ambiguous and situational.

Since good general accounts of the Substances are given elsewhere, this chapter concentrates on these areas of ambiguity and overlap that have given difficulty and confusion to Western students of TCM.

Table 3.2 outlines the principal functions and the distributions of the five main Substances, and gives their main associated Zang.

Table 3.2 The Functions of the Substances

Subsance	Main Zang Associated	Functions	Distribution
Qi	Fei, Shen Pi	moves, warms, transforms, protects, retains, & nourishes	inside & outside Jing Luo & Xue Mai
Xue	Xin, Gan Pi	nourishes & moistens	in Xue Mai & Jing Luo
Jin Ye	Shen, Fei, Pi	moistens & nourishes	throughout the Body
Jing	Shen	activates transformations, & controls growth, development & reproduction	in Eight Extra channels & in Jing Luo; stored in Shen
Shen*	Xin	vitalizes Body & consciousness	resides in Xin

Yin Yang and the Substances

The foundation of an understanding of the Substances is an understanding of Yin Yang.

Firstly, Yin Yang is relative, e.g. Jing is Yin relative to Qi, but Yang relative to Xue.

Secondly, all phenomena, whether relatively Yin or Yang, have both a Yin and Yang aspect. For example, although Qi is relatively Yang, energetic and immaterial, it can have aspects of Yang or Yin, depending on the situation, as in its sub-division into Wei Qi and Ying Qi, as shown in Table 3.3.

Table 3.3 The Yin and Yang Aspects of Qi, Jin Ye and Jing

Substance	Yang Aspect	Yin Aspect
Qi	Wei warms & protects skin, Muscles & Body surface	Ying nourishes Zang Fu & Tissues
Jin Ye	Jin moistens, warms & nourishes skin & Muscles	Ye moistens & nourishes Zang Fu, joints, Bones, Brain and Orifices
Jing	warming, energizing aspect; activates transformations, growth, development & reproduction	fluid, nourishing aspect; material basis for form- ation of Bone Marrow, Brain & Xue

Only Qi and Jin Ye have named Yin and Yang sub-divisions, those of Jing being associated with the Yin and Yang, Fire and Water aspects of Shen (Kidney). Though Xue is relatively Yin and Shen⋆ is relatively Yang, they have both Yin and Yang aspects but the division is less prominent than with Qi, Jin Ye and Jing.

Thirdly, Yin and Yang are dependent upon each other; Yin nourishes Yang, and Yang protects Yin. For example, Qi moves Xue, and Xue nourishes Qi.

Formation of the Substances

Consideration of the formation of the basic Substances, involves an understanding of Zang Fu physiology and interrelationships; this will be dealt with in greater detail in Parts II and III.

Qi

Gu Qi, derived from food and drink, by the action of Pi and Wei (Spleen and Stomach), combines in the Chest with air from Fei (Lungs) to form Zong and Zhen Qi, under the influence of Xin and Fei (Heart and Lungs). Zong Qi, the Qi of the Chest, is closely related to the functions of Xin and Fei, and their movement of Xue and Qi, respectively, around the Body.

Wei Qi and Ying Qi are the two aspects of Zhen Qi, True Qi. Wei circulates mainly in the skin and Muscles, and Ying circulates mainly in Jing Luo and Xue Mai. The nature and functions of Ying Qi and of Xue are so close that in some texts and in some situations, the two terms are synonymous.

Figure 3.1 is over-simplified and overly clear, and in some texts, the distinctions between the various categories are rather blurred, as for example between Zong Qi and Zhen Qi.

Xue

Gu Qi, derived from food and drink, is transformed to Xue in the Chest, by the action of Xin and Fei. Also, the Yin aspect of Jing, stored in Shen (Kidney), gives rise to Bone Marrow, which in turn produces Xue. Further, the Yang aspect of Jing, or Yuan Qi, activates the transformations performed by both Xin and Fei in the Upper Jiao, and Pi and Wei in the Middle Jiao.

Figure 3.1 Formation of Qi and Xue

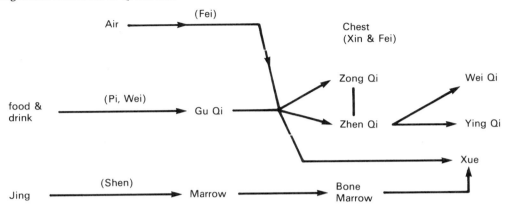

Jin Ye

Food and drink is transformed by Pi and Wei into the various denser and lighter fractions of Jin Ye (Body Fluids). Jin, the purer, lighter, more Yang and dynamic fraction, goes via Fei to warm, moisten and nourish the skin and Muscles. It has a function and distribution similar to Wei Qi. Ye is less pure, denser, more Yin and more substantial, and has a distribution similar to Ying Qi, and goes to moisten and nourish the Zang Fu, Bones, Brain and Orifices. Jin Ye circulate through the Body inside and outside Jing Luo and Xue Mai, providing moisture and nourishment to Tissues and Zang Fu.

Figure 3.2 Formation of Jin Ye

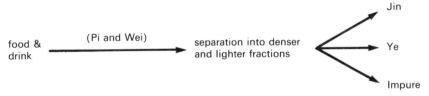

The densest fraction goes via Xiao Chang (Small Intestine), to Pang Guang (Bladder) and Da Chang (Colon), where, after some reabsorption, the relatively more fluid and relatively more solid fractions are passed from the body as urine and faeces respectively.

The terms Fluids or Body Fluids, often used as translations for Jin Ye, represent a fundamentally different concept from the body fluids of Western physiology. Ye may refer to any type of fluid, but Jin Ye refers specifically to fluids secreted by living cells, although the two terms may be used interchangeably. Jin Ye includes the secretions of the body:- tears, sweat, saliva, milk; nasal, gastric and genital secretions; and so on. However, the fluid waste, urine, is an excretion, and is considered to be Ye, not Jin Ye.

In certain contexts, for example when loosely referring to the fluid component of the Body, the terms Jin Ye and Water may be used interchangeably. However, Jin Ye refers more to the specific secretions of the Body, whereas Water is a more general and inclusive term referring to all the fluids in the Body, whether pure or impure. The term Water also has the meaning of the principle of Water, as opposed to the principle of Fire.

Jing

Terminology has been simplified here; Jing is used as a general term for a group of overlapping concepts. Prenatal Jing is derived from the Jing of the parents. Postnatal Jing is formed from the purified fraction of the transformation products of food and drink.

Figure 3.3 Formation of Jing

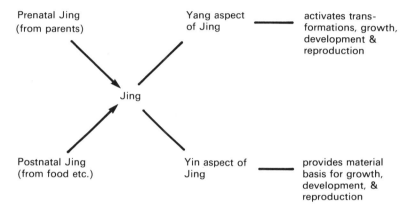

The Yang aspect of Jing, approximately corresponding to the Yang aspect of Shen (Kidney) Qi, or to Yuan Qi, is responsible for the Yang functions of warming, activating, transforming and moving; as in the transformations involved in the formation of Qi, Xue and Jin Ye, or those involved in growth, development and reproduction.

Yuan Qi is a term sometimes used more or less synonymously with the Yang aspect of Shen Jing, Shen Yang Qi, or the Fire of Ming Men. It has other attributes, but these will not be discussed here.

The Yin aspect of Jing provides a material base for the dynamic activities of the Yang aspect; indeed, the two aspects are complementary and inseparable. The Yin aspect provides the substratum for the formation of the materials associated with Jing:- Marrow, Xue, etc.

Figure 3.4 Yin Aspect of Jing

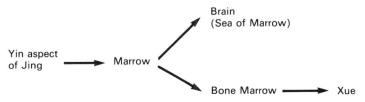

Shen

Prenatal Shen★ is derived from the parents, and Postnatal Shen★ is derived from, or is the manifestation of, the interaction of Jing and Qi. Xin Xue and Xin Yin provide the Residence for Shen★, since, in TCM, consciousness resides not so much in the Brain, as in Xin (Heart). Shen★ vitalizes the Body and consciousness, and provides the driving force behind the personality. Together, Jing, Qi and Shen★, form the San Bao, or the Three Treasures.

Figure 3.5 Formation of Shen★

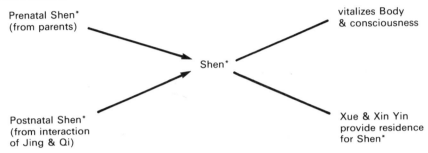

This conception of Shen★ implies a material aspect of Shen★, foreign to the Western idea of Spirit; in TCM, Shen★ is an integral part of the Body, not an entity separate from it.

Figure 3.6 summarizes the interrelations involved in the formation of Qi, Xue and Jing.

Ambiguities

Overlapping function and conceptual ambiguity can make clear understanding of the Substances difficult for Western students of TCM. The ten pairings of the five main Substances are discussed below, to clarify the similarities, differences and interrelationships between each pair.

Qi and Xue

Relatively, Qi is Yang and Xue is Yin. Traditionally, Qi is the commander of Xue, and Xue is the mother of Qi. Qi activates the formation of Xue, and moves and retains it within the vessels. Xue nourishes and moistens the Zang Fu that form and govern the Qi.

The relationship between Xue and Ying Qi, the Yin aspect of Zhen Qi, is so close that the terms Xue and Ying Qi are sometimes used interchangeably. They are both concerned with nourishment, and they move together through Xue Mai. However, within this intimate relationship, Xue is relatively Yin and substantial, and Ying is relatively Yang, immaterial and dynamic.

Qi and Jin Ye

Relatively, Qi is less substantial and more Yang than Jin Ye. Qi activates the formation and movement of Jin Ye within the Body, and Jin Ye moistens and nourishes the Zang Fu.

Figure 3.6 Formation of the Substances

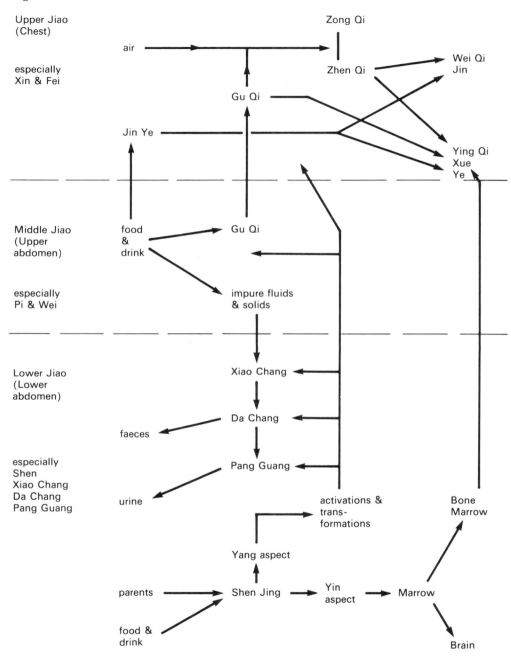

Both Jin and Wei Qi circulate outside the Jing Luo and warm, moisten and nourish the skin and Muscles. However, the emphasis of Wei Qi is on protecting the Body from outside invasion, whereas the emphasis of Jin is on moistening.

Ye and Ying Qi are relatively more Yin, and flow together to moisten and nourish Zang Fu and Tissues. However, the emphasis of Ye is on moistening, and that of Ying is on nourishment. Also, Ye has a special relationship with the Brain, Bones and Orifices.

Qi and Jing

Jing is more substantial and Yin than Qi. Prenatal and Postnatal Jing activate the formation of Qi, and Qi activates the formation of Postnatal Jing from food and drink. The relationship of Shen Qi and Shen Jing is especially close and will be discussed in Part II. Wei Qi and the Yang aspect of Jing, both move, warm and activate; Ying Qi and the Yin aspect of Jing, both have a function of nourishment. However, Jing is specifically associated with Shen (Kidneys), and with growth, development, reproduction and inheritance. The Yin aspect of Jing provides the material basis for these processes, and the Yang aspect actives them.

Qi is responsible for the day-to-day functioning of the body, but Jing is also responsible for the seven and eight year developmental cycles of TCM.

Qi and Shen*

Both are relatively Yang, Shen* being the more Yang and insubstantial. Shen* arises from the interraction of Qi and Jing, and gives the Qi of the Body the unique qualities of awareness, consciousness and vitality .

Xue and Jin Ye

Both are relatively Yin, and form part of the continuum of fluids within the Body. Xue and Jin Ye are mutually dependent. Loss of Xue will affect Jin Ye, and damage to Jin Ye, with the Yin Deficiency and Heat often asociated with it, will affect the quality and quantity of Xue. Both nourish and moisten, but Xue is more refined, and is more concerned with nourishment, and Jin Ye with moistening.

Xue and Jing

Though both are Yin relative to Qi, Jing is Yang relative to Xue. The Yin aspect of Jing provides the material base for Xue formation, and the Yang aspect activates this process. Xue nourishes and moistens the Zang Fu concerned with the formation of Postnatal Jing, including Shen, where both Prenatal and Postnatal Jing is stored.

Like Qi, Xue is involved in day-to-day metabolism, whereas Jing is also involved in the long-term cycles of development and reproduction.

Xue and Shen*

Shen* is Yang relative to Xue. Xin rules both Shen* and Xue. Xin Xue and Xin Yin provide the residence of Shen*, and if they are Deficient, Shen* will have no residence and will be disturbed. Conversely, if Shen* is disturbed, Xin function may be disturbed, leading to Xin Xue and Xin Yin Deficiencies.

Jin Ye and Jing

Both are relatively Yin, both have comparable Yin and Yang aspects, both are ruled by Shen. Jing activates the formations and transformations of Jin Ye, and Ye moistens and nourishes the Zang Fu that replenish the Jing, including Shen that stores it. There is a close association between Jing and Ye, since both are associated with Brain and Bone Marrow; Jing with their formation, and Ye with their lubrication. Both have fluid attributes, and both may moisten and nourish. However, Jing has an irreplaceable inherited component. Even Post- natal Jing is more refined then Jin Ye and it is more precious, since it is less easily replaced. Also, whereas Jin Ye is more concerned with the everyday economy of the Body, Jing is more concerned with its deeper, more fundamental rhythms.

Jin Ye and Shen★

Jin Ye are the least refined, and Shen★ the most refined of the Substances. The state of Jin Ye affects Xin Xue and Xin Yin, and hence Shen★. Conversely, disturbance of Shen★ may affect Jin Ye, via Yin and Xue.

Jing and Shen★

Shen★ is more refined and more Yang. Shen★ is the manifestation of Jing and Qi, and is ruled by Xin; Jing is ruled by Shen. The relationships of Xin and Shen, and of Shen★ and Jing, are fundamental to Chinese medicine.

In summary, there are two main groups of overlapping concepts:-

Yang Group   Wei Qi, Jin, Shen★, and the Yang aspect of Jing

Yin Group   Ying Qi, Ye, Xue, and the Yin aspect of Jing

Within each group, each Substance has functions that overlap with each of the other Substances in that group. For example, Ying Qi has functions in common with Ye, with Xue, and with the Yin aspect of Jing. In addition, each Substance has functions specific to itself alone.

Patterns of Disharmony of the Substances

The four main Patterns of Disharmony of the Substances are:-

Deficient Qi   Deficient Xue   Stagnant Qi   Stagnant Xue

Table 3.4 compares the patterns of Deficient Yang, Deficient Yin, and the four main Substance disharmonies. In addition to these six main Patterns of Disharmony, there are also the four relatively less important patterns:-

Dificient Jin Ye   Deficient Jing   Deficient Shen★   Disturbance of Shen★

Deficient Jin Ye

This category is usually included under patterns of Deficient Yin, Deficient Heat or Excess Heat. However, it is not necessarily associated with patterns of Heat, for example loss of blood, vomiting and diarrhoea, may also involve loss of Jin Ye. Signs of this Deficiency include dryness, thinness, and frequently signs of Heat.

Deficient Jing

Either or both of the Yin or Yang aspects of Jing may become Deficient, for a variety of reasons, discussed in Chapter 7 on Shen. Associated signs involve

Table 3.4 The Basic Patterns of Disharmony of the Substances

Pattern	Main Zang associated	Main Signs	Pulse	Tongue	Example
Deficient Qi	Shen, Pi, Fei	bright pale face; general weakness; weak breathing & voice	empty	pale flabby	asthma (Deficient Fei Qi & Shen Qi type)
Deficient Yang	Shen, Pi, Xin	Deficient Qi signs, but more severe; plus signs of Cold, e.g. cold limbs, aversion to cold	slow sinking	pale moist	oedema (Deficient Shen Yang & Pi Yang type)
Deficient Xue	Pi, Xin Gan	dull pale face; numbness or weak tremors in limbs; emaciation; dizziness	thin choppy	pale thin	anaemia (Deficient (Pi Qi type)
Deficient Yin	Shen, Gan, Xin, Fei	signs of Heat, e.g. restlessness, malar flush, emaciation, dizziness	thin rapid	red thin	insomnia (Deficient Shen Yin & Xin Yin type)
Stagnant Qi	Gan, Xin, Fei	distention & soreness, often of changing location	wiry tight	purple	premenstrual tension (Stagnant Qi type)
Stagnant Xue	Gan, Xin	severe pain, often of fixed location; dark complexion	choppy full	dark purple	angina pectoris (Stagnant Xin Xue type)

problems of reproduction and growth, and of Tissues relying on Jing for nourishment and formation, for example Bones, Xue, Brain, ears, etc.

Deficient Shen★

Signs of Deficient Shen★ may be associated with general Deficiency of Qi and Jing, or, more specifically, with a variety of Deficiencies of Xin. The signs include dullness, apathy, and lack of spirit, vitality, and joy.

Disturbance of Shen★

This pattern is often associated with Deficiency of Xin Yin or Deficiency of Xin Xue, or with extreme Heat and Phlegm. Signs such as restlessness, insomnia, irritability, confused speech, extreme mental disturbance, and loss of consciousness may occcur.

Further Ambiguities

A common area of confusion for Westerners lies in the overlap of the Patterns of Disharmony of Yin, Yang, Qi, and Xue, outlined in Table 3.4 above. There are four overlapping continua:-

Yin ——— Yang   Yang ——— Qi

Yin ——— Xue   Xue ——— Qi

These four continua form the basis for an understanding of Zang Fu pathology.
It is most important to be able to differentiate between the two possibilities in
each of the following five pairs of Patterns of Disharmony listed below:-

Deficient Yang   and   Deficient Yin
Deficient Qi   and   Deficient Yang
Deficient Qi   and   Deficient Xue
Deficient Xue   and   Deficient Yin
Stagnant Qi   and   Stagnant Xue

Deficient Yang and Deficient Yin
This division into Deficient Yang and Deficient Yin, is the foundation of Chinese
Pathology. Deficient Yang is associated with signs of Cold; and with an
accumulation of fluid, due to lack of Yang to move Qi and Xue, and to transform
and move Jin Ye. Deficient Yin is associated with signs of Heat; and with
Deficiency of of Jin Ye, due to lack of Yin to control the Heat, with resultant
damage to the fluids of the Body. Hence, the difference in the signs of these two
patterns as shown in Table 3.5.

Table 3.5 Comparison of the Signs of Deficient Yang and Deficient Yin

Sign	Deficient Yang	Deficient Yin
Heat-Cold	chilly	feverish
Urine	clear, copious	dark, concentrated
Faeces	loose & moist	dry & hard
Pulse	slow	rapid
Tongue	pale, moist, flabby	red, dry, thin

However, there are situations where the patient may show signs of both
Deficient Yin and Deficient Yang. This is not referring to the conditions of
Illusionary Cold and Illusionary Heat, which are very severe acute or crisis
situations, but to the less severe conditions of chronic Deficiency that form the
bulk of Western practice. There are two main origins of the simultaneous
occurrence of signs of Deficient Yin and signs of Deficient Yang:-

1.   Deficient Qi and Deficient Yin

     For example, a case where there is a Deficiency of Yin relative to Yang, but an
     overall Deficiency of Qi. Although there may be signs of Hyperactive Yang
     and the Heat in the upper Body, due to inability of Yin to control Yang, there
     is not enough Qi to perform the relatively Yang functions of activation,
     transformation and movement, resulting in lack of energy, and in chilliness,
     especially in the lower Body.

2. Deficient Yin of some Zang Fu with Deficient Yang of other Zang Fu. For example, Depression of Gan Qi aggravates a condition of Deficient Qi of Pi and Deficient Yang of Pi. However, Depression of Gan Qi may also give rise to Hyperactive Gan Yang and Blazing Gan Fire. Hence, signs of Heat and Excess may be associated with Gan, at the same time that signs of Deficiency and Cold are associated with Pi.

These two origins are often intermingled, and in such patients, sometimes Deficient Yin may predominate, and sometimes Deficient Yang, depending upon conditions. For example, in conditions of malnutrition and External Cold, Deficient Yang may predominate, whereas in conditions of External Heat and emotional stress, Deficient Yin may predominate.

Deficient Qi and Deficient Yang
Yang is a broader, more fundamental concept than Qi. The division into Yin and Yang, Fire and Water, Heat and Cold, lies at the heart of Chinese medicine. Since Qi is just one of the aspects of Yang, the signs of Yang Deficiency generally include the signs of Deficient Qi, but since Deficient Yang may also be seen as a progression of Deficient Qi, these shared signs are usually more severe in the case of Deficient Yang. In addition, Deficient Yang has signs of Cold and Damp.

Deficient Qi and Deficient Xue
The Qi-Xue relationship has already been discussed. Due to the nourishing function of both Xue and Ying Qi, Deficiency of both Qi and Xue will lead to weakness of Body and pulse, and to paleness of face and tongue. However, due to the relationship of Qi with Yang, and of Xue with Yin, Deficiency of Qi often has signs of Cold, whereas Deficient Xue often has signs of Dryness. Hence Deficiency of Xue may have the thin emaciated body, thin pulse, thin tongue, dry skin and dry hair, associated with reduction of fluids. Nevertheless, Deficient Qi and Deficient Xue commonly occur together, especially in cases of chronic debility.

Deficient Xue and Deficient Yin
The relationship between Deficient Xue and Deficient Yin is not the same as that between Deficient Qi and Deficient Yang. There is an intimate association between Yin, Xue and Jin Ye, so that both Deficient Yin and Deficient Xue have signs of dryness. However, although Deficient Xue is often associated with Deficient Yin and signs of Heat, this is not necessarily the case; indeed, a common distinction between the two patterns is the presence of or absence of signs of Heat.

Although Yin and Xue form a continuum, there is a qualitative difference between them, greater than the difference between Qi and Yang. Also, although Xue and Yin share some signs, for example those due to the reduction of fluids, Deficient Yin does not tend to include all the signs of Deficient Xue, as Deficient Yang includes the signs of Deficient Qi. Nor is Deficient Yin necessarily a progression of Deficient Xue, nor is Deficient Yin a much deeper pathological phenomenon than Deficient Xue, although Deficient Yin is a more fundamental concept, with a broader application.

Stagnant Qi and Stagnant Xue
Stagnant Qi and Stagnant Xue may have common origins, and the latter is often a progression of the former, especially in the sense of increased severity and immobility of signs. For example, since Stagnant Xue is more material than Stagnant Qi, if there are palpable lumps these are harder and more persistent, than in the case of Stagnant Qi. Also, whilst with Stagnant Qi, there is distension and soreness, which may come and go and change location, Stagnant Xue is characterized by severe pain which is stabbing, constant and of fixed location. Since obstruction is more material and more constant in the case of Stagnant Xue, the pulse is fuller, and the tongue and complexion darker.

Summary

An understanding of the nature, physiology, pathology, and interrelationships of the Substances is basic to an understanding of Zang Fu. This Chapter has briefly considered the five basic Substances of TCM, their formation and Patterns of Disharmony, in terms of Yin Yang and of Zang Fu. Areas of ambiguity and overlap have been discussed; especially between the different pairs of Substances, and between the different pairs of Patterns of Disharmony of the Substances.

Chapter

4

Origins of Disease

The three basic components of disease are the Body, the Disease Factors, and the Pattern of Disharmony. These three are so closely interwoven that they are really inseparable, but they can be arbitrarily represented:-

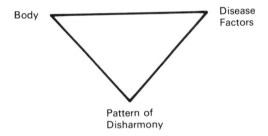

The Disease Factors are the originating or precipitating factors associated with the Origin of the illness. The Pattern of Disharmony is the complex of internal pathological changes and external signs associated with this particular imbalance in the interaction between the Body and the environment. The Body is the foundation for the physical, emotional, mental and spiritual life of the individual; and is based on an organizational framework of Substances, Jing Luo, Zang Fu and Tissues.

Origins of Disease

The Western and the Chinese approaches to the Origins of Disease are very different. Harmony is the ultimate goal within Chinese mysticism, philosophy, culture and medicine; harmony within the individual, between the individual and the natural world, and between the individual and society. Chinese thought sees the disease as Disharmony; as a disharmonious pattern in the interaction between the Body and the environment. Therefore, Chinese medicine aims at the accurate perception, classification and treatment of Patterns of Disharmony, in order to restore harmony to the individual.

Western medicine tends to see disease in terms of biochemistry and bacteriology, not in terms of the harmony of the individual. It generally attempts to isolate a single cause from a linear chain of cause and effect; and to treat this single cause, rather than treat the patient as a whole. In contrast to this reductive approach, TCM attempts to synthesize as complete a pattern as possible, and does not strongly differentiate between cause and effect. Also, TCM does not think so much in terms of causes, as in terms of Disease Factors, factors that are associated with the origination or precipitation of disease. Again, it does not think in terms of a single factor, but in terms of a number of contributing factors. Especially, it views all the Disease Factors, all the internal pathological changes and external signs of disharmony, and the Body itself, as being integral parts of an overall pattern.

The Western and Chinese approaches can be contrasted as follows:-

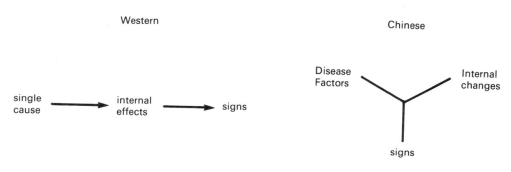

For example, in the Western approach:-

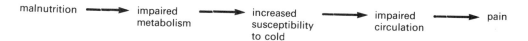

whereas in the Chinese approach:-

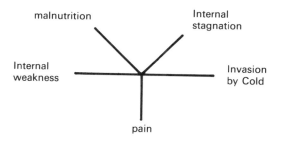

This account exaggerates the differences between Western and Chinese medicine. In some areas, the Western approach to disease is more sophisticated than is outlined above; and there are hints of causality in Chinese medicine.

Disease Factors

Disease Factors are factors associated with the origin of disharmony in the Body. TCM considers three main groups of Disease Factors, as shown in Table 4.1. The interrelationship between the individual and the environment may be arbitrarily divided into factors that are External, arising from the environment; Internal, arising within the Body; and Miscellaneous, partaking of both Body and environment. These three categories approximate to:- climate, emotions, and lifestyle (Table 4.2).

Table 4.1 Classification of Disease Factors

External Disease Factors	Internal Disease Factors	Disease Factors Neither Internal nor External (Miscellaneous)
Wai Yin	Nei Yin	Bu Nei Wai Yin

Table 4.2 List of Main Disease Factors in TCM

Climate	Emotions	Lifestyle
Six Pernicious Influences (Liu Yin)	Seven Emotions (Qi Qing)	Miscellaneous (Bu Nei Wai Yin)
Wind	Joy	Nutrition
Cold	Anger	Occupation
Heat	Pensiveness	Overwork
Damp	Sorrow	Exercise
Dryness	Fear	Relationships
Summer Heat	Fright	Sex
	Grief	Trauma
		Parasites

External Factors

TCM regards climate as the most important External source of potential Disease Factors. Climate is composed of six basic climatic phenomena, or environmental factors:- Wind, Cold, Heat, Damp, Dryness, and Summer Heat. Fluctuation of the levels of these factors within moderate limits is a natural part of a healthy life.

When these factors are in Excess, they may become Liu Yin, variously translated as the Six Climatic Aberrations, the Six Pernicious Influences, the Six Excesses, the Six External Disease Factors, and so on. In this book, they will be referred to mainly as the External Disease Factors. An alternative Chinese term is Liu Xie. Xie may be translated as incorrect, improper, wayward, evil, or devilish. Hence, Liu Xie may be interpreted as the Six Evils or the Six Devils.

In TCM, there is the important concept of Yu or impediment. As long as there is an adequate, unobstructed flow of Qi and Xue, there can be no illness in the Body. Once there is an impediment to this flow, illness occurs.

Generally, if the Body is healthy and strong, Yin and Yang are in balance, Qi is sufficient, and the Body is not affected by fluctuations in the climatic factors, unless these are both extreme and prolonged. If, however, there is Internal disharmony, and the Body, especially Wei Qi, is weakened, climatic factors may be able to invade the Body, and are then termed Pernicious Influences. A climatic factor only becomes a Pernicious Influence, when it is involved in originating disharmony within the Body.

If the weakness of the Body and Wei Qi is only mild, the struggle between Pernicious Influence and Wei Qi results in expulsion of Pernicious Influence and recovery of the patient. However, if the Deficiency of Wei Qi is pronounced, and the Pernicious Influence extreme, Wei Qi may fail to expel the Pernicious Influence, which may then go deeper into the Body, so that the illness becomes more serious, recovery is delayed, and convalescence prolonged. In TCM, treatment aims at assisting the Body to disperse and expel the External Disease Factors, in cases where these have invaded and lodged in the Body.

The term Excess, with respect to a climatic factor, is relative; for example, one person may withstand extreme levels of Heat, which in another person would precipitate illness, and yet the second person might withstand extreme levels of Damp, which in the first person might originate disharmony.

Also, the distinction between External Disease Factors and Internal Disease Factors often becomes blurred. For example, Wind, Cold, Heat, Damp and Dryness, may arise both Externally, as climatic factors, or Internally, associated with Internal disharmony. In diagnosis, it is most important to distinguish, for example, Internal Heat from External Heat, since they represent different Patterns of Disharmony, requiring different treatment. Differentiation is made according to the signs of disharmony; for example, the External Heat Pattern may be associated with recent exposure to External Heat, and with acute illness; the Internal Heat Pattern may be associated with more chronic illness, and with signs of long-term disharmony of one or more Zang Fu.

Furthermore, one Liu Xie may transform into another. For example, once it has invaded the Body, External Wind Cold may transform into Heat; Internal Damp may give rise to Internal Damp Heat, or to Internal Fire; and both External and Internal Cold and Damp may give rise to Stagnation and Phlegm, the two secondary Disease Factors mentioned on page 44, and discussed in detail in later chapters.

Wind

Wind, the climatic factor, is a normal part of the natural environment. When the Body is weak, if Wind the climatic factor is in relative Excess, it may enter and injure the Body, and is then termed Wind the Pernicious Influence.

Wind may also be considered as any sudden change of climate; and is often closely associated with other factors, such as Cold, Heat, Damp and Dryness, potentiating their effects, and enabling them to invade the Body more easily. TCM recognizes such combinations of Disease Factors as Wind Cold, Wind Heat, Wind Damp, Wind Dryness and Wind Phlegm.

As wind in nature moves the leaves and branches of a tree, so Wind in the Body may affect the Body parts and functions.

Wind is characterized by constant movement, and the effects of pathogenic Wind in the Body include abnormal movement or rigidity of head, limbs or trunk, such as numbness, spasms, tremors and convulsions.

Since Wind is light and Yang, it tends to affect the top of the Body, especially the head, neck and face; and to affect the outermost parts of the Body, especially the skin and muscles.

In Five Phase Theory, Wind is associated with spring, but the phenomena of External Wind and Internal Wind are not limited to this season. Sudden changes of weather, or winds as such, may occur at any time of the year. Spring and Autumn are especially changeable, but there are often sudden warm spells in winter, and sudden cold spells in summer.

External Wind

The Body may be invaded by External Wind, following a sudden change in climate; by exposure to wind, especially after perspiring; or by sitting or sleeping in a draught.

The signs of invasion by External Wind are often of sudden onset, with fever, sweating, aversion to wind, headache, nasal obstruction, sore or itchy throat, superficial pulse, and tongue with thin coat. This roughly corresponds to the early stages of infections or contagious diseases in Western Medicine, such as the common cold and influenza.

Table 4.3 Signs and Pathology of External Wind

Signs	Pathology
fear of wind	failure of Wei Qi to warm skin and muscles
fever	struggle between Wei Qi and pathological Wind
perspiration	weakness of Wei Qi allows opening of the pores
nasal congestion ⎫	Wind tends to invade Fei, which governs the nose
itchy throat ⎭	and throat
headache	Wind invasion of Jing Luo of the head, especially Tai Yang, disturbs the circulation of Qi
superficial pulse	effects of Wind invasion are mainly at the surface of the Body

External Wind tends to affect the uppermost and outermost parts of the Body. Since Fei is considered to be the Yin organ system in most direct contact with the external environment, it is the Zang most commonly invaded by Wind; especially by Wind Cold and Wind Heat, which may transform into one another.

Internal Wind

Both Internal and External Wind are light and Yang, and tend to affect the upper part of the body, especially the head, neck and face. However, they have different origins and different signs, and do not generally give rise to each other. Where External Wind results from the exposure of a weakened Body to sudden draughts or changes in climate, Internal Wind arises from a variety of different causes, including Deficient Xue, high fevers, and Hyperactive Gan Yang. Internal Wind is discussed in Chapter 9, pages 113-118.

Just as the Zang most associated with External Wind is Fei, Internal Wind is closely associated with disharmony of Gan. Internal Wind represents sudden irregular movement, the opposite of the smooth even flow of Qi promoted by Gan. These rapid gusts of upward movement disturb the movement of Qi and Xue in the Jing Luo, and may be accompanied by tics, tremors, spasms, convulsions, dizziness or loss of consciousness.

Table 4.4 Comparison of the Signs of External Wind and Internal Wind

External Wind	Common Signs	Internal Wind
fear of wind stuffy nose itchy throat superficial pulse	often sudden onset signs may come and go signs may change location upper body especially affected	dizziness numbness of limbs tremors, convulsions loss of consciousness, often wiry pulse

External Wind is associated with the early stages of infectious diseases, whereas Internal Wind may be associated with such disorders as high fevers, facial tremors, and cerebrovascular accidents and their sequellae. Both External Wind and some forms of Internal Wind may be accompanied by fever, but at the opposite extremes of the scale. External Wind may be associated with relatively mild fever, at superficial depth in the Body, corresponding to the Tai Yang stage of Cold Diseases. In contrast, Internal Wind, of the type associated with Utmost Heat, may relate to the deepest, most serious stage of fever, the Ying stage of the Warm Disease classification.

Relationships to other Factors

External Wind may potentiate the effects of Cold in the Body, and the two factors may be very closely related. However, the signs associated with Wind may be differentiated from those associated with Cold:-

Table 4.5 Comparison of the Signs of External Wind and External Cold

External Wind	Common Signs	External Cold
aversion to Wind perspiration no shortness of breath pulse not tight	fear of wind and cold fever headache superficial pulse	aversion to cold no perspiration shortness of breath pulse tight

Similarly, the signs of External Wind Cold can be differentiated from the signs of External Wind Heat:-

Table 4.6 Comparison of the Signs of Wind Cold and Wind Heat

Wind Cold	Common Signs	Wind Heat
more chills than fever less perspiration tight superficial pulse tongue coat white	fever and chills perspiration superficial pulse thin tongue coat	more fever than chills more perspiration rapid superficial pulse tongue coat yellow

External Wind may potentiate or combine with External Cold, Heat, Damp and Dryness. Internal Wind may combine especially with Phlegm and Fire, as discussed on page 116; and Internal Heat in Xue may combine with External Wind, and manifest in red and itchy skin eruptions.

Cold

Whereas Wind is a Yang phenomenon, Cold is a Yin factor, and tends to depress the Yang of the Body, specifically the Yang functions of warming, moving, transforming, retaining and protecting.

Table 4.7 Signs Associated with Depression of the Yang Functions by Cold

Yang Functions	Effect of Cold
warming	person feels cold
moving	Stagnation of movement of Qi, leading to pain
transformation	Deficiency of the Substances and incomplete digestion
retaining	loss of fluids, e.g. more copious urination or nasal secretions
protecting	insufficient Wei Qi and Ying Qi at the Body surface, with easier entry of External Disease Factors

Both in nature and in the Body, Cold slows activity and movement. In the Body, it contracts the Jing Luo, with the retardation, obstruction and stagnation of the flow of Qi and Xue, and severe pain relieved by warmth and aggravated by cold.

Cold, and the diseases associated with Cold are related to Winter. However, just as Wind may occur in any season, so the Body may be invaded by External Cold at any time of the year.

External Cold

Signs of Cold may follow exposure to cold weather, especially after perspiration while wearing insufficient clothing; prolonged contact with cold water; standing on cold surfaces; or consumption of cold food and drink.

Which part of the Body is most affected by Cold will partly depend on which part of the Body is most exposed, and partly upon which part already has a stagnation in the flow of Qi, due to previous injury or predisposition.

The degree to which the Body is affected by Cold will depend partly on the severity of the Cold, and partly on the degree of weakness of the Body. As with External Wind, the penetration of the External Cold is inwards, through the outer energy layer surrounding the body, through the skin, the Muscle channels, and the muscles and flesh, before penetrating the Main channels and the deeper tissues such as the bones and joints.

The signs of External Cold are:- the patient feels cold, chills and mild fever, fear of cold and preference for warmth, severe pain relieved by warmth and aggravated by cold, little or no perspiration, general ache, lumbago and arthralgia, shortness of breath, copious clear excretions and secretions, slow, light pulse, and tongue with thin white coat.

External Cold tends to depress Yang, and since Shen Yang is the source of all

Yang in the Body, it tends to depress Shen Yang. This tends to affect those organ systems which are prone to Deficient Yang, and which therefore are reliant on Shen Yang.

Deficient Shen Yang may be aggravated by exposure to Cold of the Body in general, or of the lumbar area in particular. It may manifest especially as copious urination.

Deficient Pi Yang may be aggravated by Deficient Shen Yang, by exposure of the abdomen to Cold, or by the consumption of cold or raw food and drink. Common signs are abdominal distension, and diarrhoea with undigested food in the stools.

Deficient Xin Yang may be aggravated by Deficient Shen Yang and by exposure of the Body to Cold. This may lead to Stagnation of Xin Xue, with pain in the heart region.

Deficient Fei Yang may be aggravated by Deficient Shen Yang, and by exposure of the lungs to cold air. Signs include shortness of breath, coughing and asthma, as well as clear nasal discharge. Also, since the Cold depresses the Dispersing function of Fei, the distribution of Wei Qi and Ying Qi to the surface of the Body may be impaired, contributing to the fear of cold and the coldness of the surface of the Body.

Table 4.8 Signs and Pathology of External Cold

Signs	Pathology
feels cold, fears cold seeks warmth	reduction of Yang function of warming; failure of Ying Qi to nourish superficial part of Body; hindrance of Wei Qi by pathological Cold
mild fever and chills	attempt of Body to expel External Cold; struggle between Qi and Cold - the antipathological and pathological factors
severe pain relieved by warmth and aggravated by Cold general ache, arthralgia and lumbago	reduction of Yang function of movement; stagnation of circulation of Qi and Xue.
little or no perspiration	Cold contracts and obstructs the pores
headache	retardation of Qi circulation in Tai Yang channels
shortness of breath	Cold depresses the Dispersing and Descending functions of Fei
copious clear secretions & excretions	Cold depresses Yang function of retaining and reduces the proper Transformation and Transportation of Jin Ye
slow tight pulse	Cold reduces movement and contracts and tightens
tongue with thin white coat	tongue coat is thin since the illness is recent, and white since there is absence of Heat

Internal Cold

External Cold arises from exposure of the weakened Body to cold in the environment. Internal Cold arises from Deficient Yang, specifically Deficient Shen Yang, and the latter may enable External Cold to enter the Body more readily. External and Internal Cold may also merge together. These relationships are summarized in Figure 4.1.

Figure 4.1 Deficient Shen Yang and External and Internal Cold

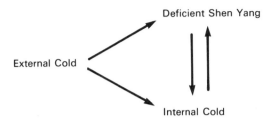

Since the Body must generally be weakened for External Cold to enter in the first place, and since prolonged External Cold may lead to Deficient Yang and hence to Internal Cold, the borderline between External and Internal Cold is rather arbitrary. However, the signs of the two patterns are differentiated in Table 4.9.

Table 4.9 Comparison of Signs of External Cold and Internal Cold

External Cold	Common Signs	Internal Cold
chills and fever	feels cold, fear of Cold	no fever
acute		chronic
superficial tight pulse	tight pulse	deep tight pulse
thin white tongue coat	white tongue coat	thick white tongue coat

Relationship with Other External Factors
External Cold and External Wind are very closely associated. Wind tends to increase the effects of Cold, both as a cooling breeze in summer or a biting icy wind in winter. The relationship between Cold and Damp is discussed later in this chapter.

Heat and Fire
The term Fire has two meanings:-

1. The Internal Evil
2. The Normal Fire of the Body
   a. Fire as opposed to Water
   b. Fire as one of the Five Phases

These two meanings of the word Fire, referring to the pathological and the physiological respectively, should not be confused.

The term Heat indicates an Evil, either External or Internal. In the sense of an Internal Evil, the terms Heat and Fire may be used interchangeably, or the use of one term or the other may depend upon the situation and upon convention. Fire sometimes refers to extreme Heat.

Heat is a Yang Evil, and is associated with summer in Five Phase Theory, but may occur in any season, especially in those predisposed to this condition. It tends to rise and affect the upper Body. It tends to damage Yin, and hence the Yin functions of cooling, moistening, nourishing and resting.

Table 4.10 Signs Associated with Damage of Yin Functions by Heat

Yin Function	Effect of Heat
cooling	signs of Heat, e.g. fever
moistening	signs of Dryness, e.g. thirst,
nourishing	signs of weakness, e.g. post-febrile debility
resting	signs of overactivity, e.g. insomnia

The effect of Heat upon the Substances and their circulation is:-

1. To damage Yin and dry up the fluids, resulting in reduced, darker, thick or sticky secretions and excretions.

2. To damage Yin, resulting in Disturbance of Shen★, with insomnia, restlessness, over-excitability and delirium.

3. To lead to 'reckless movement' of Xue, with haemorrhage and skin eruptions.

The Zang Fu which are prone to Deficient Yin are those prone to the effects of Heat and Fire. The basis of all Deficient Yin is Deficient Shen Yin, and those Zang Fu likely to be affected by this pattern are Gan, Xin, Fei and Wei.

Deficient Shen Yin is associated with reduced fluids and scanty dark urine; Deficient Gan Yin is associated with hyperactivity of Gan Yang and Gan Fire, and hence with headaches and anger; Deficient Xin Yin is associated with Disturbance of Shen★, and hence with confused speech and anxiety; Deficient Fei Yin is associated with inflammation in the lungs, and hence with dry cough, perhaps with haemoptysis; and Deficient Wei Yin is associated with irritation of the stomach, and hence with dry vomiting.

External Heat
The pattern of External Heat may arise from exposure of the Body to environmental heat, and corresponds to the Wei stage in the Wei Qi Ying Xue classification of Warm Diseases. It also corresponds to the relatively early stages of infectious febrile diseases in Western Medicine.

The signs of External Heat are high fever, patient feels hot, fear of heat, preference for cold, thirst, dry mouth, preference for cool drinks, swollen sore throat, dark scanty urine, constipation, face and body red, red skin eruptions, perhaps haemoptysis, insomnia and irritability, perhaps delirium, rapid pulse and red tongue with yellow coat.

Internal Heat
Internal Heat is associated with disturbance of the balance of Yin Yang within the Body, or within one or more organs in particular. It is associated with the patterns of Deficient Yin discussed above. Prolongued External Heat may eventually lead to Deficient Shen Yin, which in turn may lead to Internal Heat, which may then further damage Shen Yin, which will increase the effect of External Heat upon the Body.

Table 4.11 Signs and Pathology of External Heat

Signs	Pathology
feels hot, fears heat, seeks cold, fever	hyperactivity of Heat in the Body
perspiration	fluids forced out by Heat
thirst, dry mouth, scanty urine, constipation	consumption of fluids by Heat
face and body red, red skin eruptions, haemorrhage	reckless movement of Xue associated with Heat in Xue
insomnia, irritability	Disturbance of Shen* associated with the damage of Yin by Heat
rapid pulse	hyperactivity of Heat in the Body
red tongue with thin yellow coat	effect of Heat upon Xue in tongue and effect of Heat upon digestion

Figure 4.2 Deficient Shen Yin and External and Internal Heat

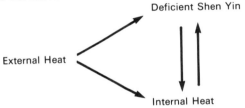

As with External and Internal Cold, the borderline between External and Internal Heat is rather vague and artificial.

Table 4.12 Comparison of Signs of External Heat and Internal Heat

External Heat	Common Signs	Internal Heat
Fever with fear of wind more recent illness superficial rapid pulse tongue with thin yellow coat	fever rapid pulse red tongue with yellow coat	higher fever less recent illness full rapid pulse redder tongue with thicker yellow coat

In Table 4.12 the Internal Heat pattern is simply the progression of the External Heat Pattern into a deeper level of the Body. The Heat is more severe and has been in the Body longer. This is an Excess Internal Heat pattern, and should not be confused with the Deficient Internal Heat patterns associated with Deficient Yin of one or more of the Zang Fu.

Relationships with other Factors
External Wind and External Heat may be closely associated, and External Wind may transform to Heat within the Body. Both Heat and Wind are Yang phenomena tending to rise up the body and be associated with rapid disturbed movement of Qi and Xue within the channels. Wind is more mobile and Internal

Wind may arise as a result of Internal Heat and Fire, just as a fire creates a draught in the natural world. Both Wind and Fire may be associated with Disturbance of Shen*, and with disorder of the circulation in the channels of the head.

Heat and Cold are facets of Fire and Water, themselves aspects of Yin and Yang, and both External and Internal Heat and Cold are closely associated with the relative Deficiencies of Yin and Yang within the Body.

Damp

Like Cold, Damp is a Yin factor; and also like Cold, it is related to the slowing, restriction, retardation and stagnation of the circulation of Qi and Jin Ye.
However, although both Cold and Damp are associated with pain, arising from the obstruction of Qi flow, Cold pain is sharp, severe and cramping, whilst Damp pain is more dull and lingering with feelings of heaviness.

There may be feelings of dullness and heaviness of the head, as if it were tightly bandaged, or in a sack; there may be fullness in the chest and epigastrium; the limbs may feel heavy, stiff and sore; and there may be a general feeling of lassitude.

Unlike Wind, which is light and Yang and tends to affect the upper parts of the Body, Damp is heavy and Yin and tends to affect the lower parts of the Body first. Also unlike Wind which is often associated with signs that come and go and move from place to place, Damp is accompanied by signs that are lingering and of fixed location.

Pathogenic Damp is also turbid and foul in nature, arising from stagnation and giving rise to it. Signs of Damp may include skin diseases, ulcers and abscesses with oozing discharge, turbid urine, diarrhoea, and heavy purulent leucorrhoea with a foul odour.

External Damp

In TCM, Damp is associated with the late summer rainy season, but may arise in any season, especially in individuals who are prone to its effects. Living in humid climates, working in water or in misty areas, living in damp rooms, wearing clothes moist with rain or perspiration, or sitting or lying on damp ground, may all result in invasion of the Body by External Damp.

Damp is Yin, and tends to depress the Yang functions of movement and transformation of the Substances, especially of Qi and Jin Ye. Among the Zang Fu, Damp tends to depress Pi function, and if the Body is exposed to External Damp and Cold for prolonged periods, Shen and Pi Yang may become weakened.

Signs of External Damp may include aversion to Damp, lethargy, feelings of heaviness in head or limbs, feelings of fullness in chest or abdomen, loss of appetite, nausea, indigestion, diarrhoea, abdominal oedema, cloudy urine, vaginal discharge, fluid-filled skin eruptions, slippery pulse and tongue with thick white, greasy coat.

Internal Damp

Internal Damp is associated with the accumulation and stagnation of fluids that may accompany the patterns of Deficient Pi Qi, Deficient Pi Yang and Deficient Shen Yang. Internal Damp may obstruct the circulation in Jing Luo, facilitating the invasion of the Body by External Damp; or over a period of time, External Damp may accumulate within the Body, damage Shen and Pi Yang, and merge with Internal Damp.

36

Table 4.13 Signs and Pathology of External Damp

Signs	Pathology
lethargy	Damp depresses Pi function, with Deficiency of Qi and Xue. Damp is turbid and lingering and obstructs free movement of Qi and Xue in Jing Luo
feelings of heaviness in head or limbs, feeling of fullness in chest or abdomen, aversion to damp	Damp is heavy and slow and dulls the circulation of Qi and Xue in Jing Luo of head, limbs, chest and abdomen
loss of appetite, nausea indigestion, diarrhoea	Damp depresses the Pi function of digestion
cloudy urine, incomplete urination, abdominal oedema, leucorrhoea, fluid-filled skin eruptions	Damp is associated with Depression of Pi function of Transformation and Transportation of Jin Ye, with obstruction and accumulation of turbid fluids
slippery pulse	represents Damp and Phlegm in the Body
tongue with thick greasy coat	represents depression of Pi function, with accumulation of Damp or Phlegm

Figure 4.3 Pi and Shen Deficiency and External and Internal Heat

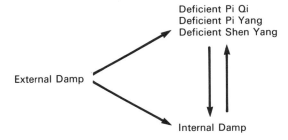

The signs of External Damp and Internal Damp are compared in Table 4.14:

Table 4.14 Comparison of Signs of External Damp and Internal Damp

External Damp	Common Signs	Internal Damp
	feelings of fullness and heaviness slippery pulse greasy tongue coat	
thinner tongue coat acute following exposure to External Damp		thicker tongue coat chronic following exposure to External Damp

Relationships with Other Factors

Damp is often associated with Cold (Damp Cold) and with Heat (Damp Heat). If the Body tends to Deficient Yang, then the depression by Damp of the Yang function of movement of Qi, may be associated with Internal Cold. Alternatively, the external environment may be both Damp and Cold, and these factors may invade the Body together.

However, long accumulation of Damp may give rise to Heat, and the phenomenon of Damp Heat. Although this may occur more readily in an individual tending to Deficient Yin and to Internal Heat, it may also occur in persons tending to Deficient Qi and Deficient Yang, in local areas of the Body where Damp has long accumulated. In fact, Deficiency of Qi is associated with poor circulation of Qi, which contributes to local stagnation and accumulation of Damp, which may become Damp Heat.

The signs of Damp, Cold, Heat, Damp Cold and Damp Heat are differentiated in Table 4.15:

Table 4.15 Comparison of Signs of Damp, Cold, Heat, Damp Cold and Damp Heat

Signs	Cold	Damp Cold	Damp	Damp Heat	Heat
feelings	of cold	of cold & heaviness or fullness	of heaviness & fullness	of heat & heaviness or fullness	of heat
pulse	slow tight	slippery slow	slippery	slippery rapid	rapid
tongue coat	white	white greasy	greasy	yellow greasy	yellow

Accumulation of Damp associated with Deficiency of Pi may give rise to Phlegm. The relationship of fluids, Pi, Damp and Phlegm is discussed on pages 84-86; and the relationships of Phlegm and Damp with Cold and heat are summarized in Figure 8.1.

Phlegm is heavier, thicker and more solid than Damp, and this is reflected in the differences in the signs of the two patterns, as summarized in Table 4.16. For example, Damp is associated with feelings of fullness and heaviness, but Phlegm may form actual lumps and tumours.

Table 4.16 Comparison of Signs of Damp and Phlegm

Damp	Common Signs	Phlegm
	Signs of Pi disharmony slippery pulse greasy tongue coat	
feelings of fullness and heaviness in limbs & trunk		lumps and nodules
feelings of heaviness in head		severe dizziness
cloudy secretions		sputum

Dryness

Traditionally, invasion of the Body by External Dryness was said to happen, in China, in the dry atmosphere of late autumn. Clinically, External Dryness is not an important factor, and Internal Dryness is not usually considered as a separate category, but included in the patterns of Heat and Deficient Yin.

Dryness is a Yang factor, and injures Yin and fluids. Signs of dryness are rough, dry, chapped skin; dry nose, mouth, lips and tongue; dry, sore throat with dry cough and little sputum; and dry stools.

Both Heat and Dryness are Yang and injure Yin and fluids, and often occur together. Heat may have signs of Dryness, but in addition may have signs such as redness, fever, perspiration, and feelings of heat. Heat is much the more important of the two patterns.

Fei is prone to invasion by External Dryness, which may manifest as dry cough with no or scanty sputum, dry nose and throat, and possible pain or difficulty of breathing; as described on page 144. The effect of External Dryness may be potentiated by External Wind, which will increase the drying effect; or by the pattern of Deficient Yin which is accompanied by Deficiency of fluids.

Summer heat

Traditionally, Summer Heat is an External factor only, that occurs solely in summer. It may be associated with prolonged exposure to the heat of the sun, or by staying in a hot room with inadequate ventiliation. However, it would be hard to separate this effect from that of working in a hot environment, for example a furnace, in a season other than summer. In other words, the same conditions might be alternatively described as External Heat or Summer Heat.

Summer Heat is a Yang factor which is said to consume Qi and Yin, and Disturb Shen*. Signs may be sudden high fever, excessive perspiration, red dry skin, restlessnes, lassitude, thirst, shortness of breath, and concentrated urine. In severe cases, there may be sudden delirium or loss of consciousness.

Summer Heat is said to have an upward direction, and a dispersive, expansive nature. Li Shi Zhen states that it can scatter the Qi, and that the pulse may become empty.

Summary

The effects of the Six Pernicious Influences in the Body resemble the effects of the six climatic factors in the external environment, the world of nature. For example, Cold is associated with the slowing of movement and the reduction of activity in both the Body and the outside world. In the winter seasons, the energies of nature and of the Body go deeper in, and there is less external activity; this is the season of rest and of storage, and of cold.

In TCM, each of the Six Pernicious Influences is seen not so much as a cause, with specific signs for its effects, but as an integral part of an overall pattern. For example, Heat is not the **cause** of the disharmony, it is a **part** of the disharmony, as are the internal pathological changes, the externally observable signs, and the functional framework of the Body itself. Indeed, all these components of the pattern of disharmony are so closely associated as to be inseparable. A pre-existing Internal disharmony may facilitate invasion of the Body by an External factor, which may then aggravate that Internal disharmony. The situation is not so much a linear chain of cause and effect, or even a 'vicious circle', it is more the simultaneous occurrence of phenomena interwoven into a pattern.

Internal Factors

These refer specifically to Qi Qing, the Seven Emotions:- joy, anger, pensiveness, sorrow, fear, fright and grief.

Emotional imbalance affects the harmonious function of the Zang Fu, the formation of the Substances, and their transportation through the Jing Luo, to all parts of the Body.

The Seven Emotions, the Five Feelings, and their relationship to the Five Zang, and to the Origins of Disease, are discussed in greater detail in Chapter 15.

Miscellaneous Factors

Bu Nei Wai Yin, the Disease Factors that are neither Internal nor External, otherwise known as the Miscellaneous Disease Factors, include:- nutrition, occupation, overwork, exercise, relationships, sex, trauma and parasites. All these categories include aspects of both Body and environment. For example, trauma and parasites may involve factors from the external environment, but may arise from Internal disharmony resulting in careless behaviour.

Constitution

The constitution may be defined as the general level of health and strength of the Body at any given time. The constitution results from the continuous interaction between the inherited genetic make-up of the individual and the environment.

Dr Shen (24) divides life into three parts:- life before birth, childhood, and adult life.

Life Before Birth

This period of life can be influenced by various factors:-

1.   The state of the Jing of the parents, prior to conception
2.   The state of the mother during pregnancy
3.   Events during birth

Disease may originate in one or more of these three main areas. The Jing of one or both parents may be Deficient, so that the sperm and/or ovum are weakened; the mother may be ill, malnourished, emotionally disturbed, or taking drugs during pregnancy; and the birth may be abnormal, difficult and prolonged. Hence, the baby may be born with illness or the predisposition to illness. This predisposition may be to general weakness, to particular types of emotional or mental imbalance, or to diseases of particular Zang Fu or of particular areas of the Body.

Childhood

The subconscious mind of an infant is an almost clean slate, and is extremely impressionable to negative as well as to positive influences. Childhood is the time when negative experiences can etch themselves into the subconscious more deeply than in later life. Also, this is the time of greatest physical growth and development, when certain pressures on the physical body can have great and lasting effect; for example malnutrition, trauma and excess sex.

Adult Life

Although less impressionable than childhood, adult life is longer, and the adult less resilient than the child to shocks and illness. Problems must be dealt with as they arise, or they will both weaken the Body and embed themselves into it.

Generally, if the constitution has been poor since birth, or if the specific disease has been present since that time, the prognosis is poor. If the problem is only recent, or has only occurred during adult life, the prognosis is more favourable. There are, however, may cases of individuals who have had difficult births and sickly childhoods, but who have later overcome these difficulties and had strong and healthy adult lives.

Nutrition

Nutritional problems arise in three main categories:-

    (i)   Malnutrition
        Deficient intake of basic requirements due to poverty, ignorance or folly; or impaired digestion, absorption and metabolism.
    (ii)   Excess
        Excessive intake of food in general, or of certain foods in particular, expecially of those foods which are particularly harmful in excess.
    (iii) Unwise Eating Habits
        Eating at irregular intervals, oscillation from extremes of feasting to extremes of fasting, eating whilst hurried or emotionally upset, etc.

The effects of nutritional imbalance are generally either Yin, associated with Cold, and often with Deficiency; or Yang, associated with Heat, and often with Excess.

Yin Effects

Insufficiency of food and drink may lead to Deficient Pi Qi, and to Deficient Qi, Deficient Xue, and Deficient Postnatal Jing. Excessive Intake of cold or raw food and drink may lead to Deficient Pi Yang, Retention of Fluid in Wei due to Cold, and Invasion of Pi by Cold and Damp.

Yang Effects

Overeating, or excessive intake of rich greasy fatty foods, sugary foods, contaminated foods, or alcohol may lead to Retention of Food in Wei, Blazing Wei Fire, Accumulation of Damp Heat in Pi, Damp Heat Invading Da Chang, Damp Heat in Gan and Dan, and Blazing Gan Fire.

Occupation

Occupational problems arise in two main categories:-

    (i)   Physical
        Many occupations have their characteristic hazards to health. For example: the prolonged slouched-seated posture of clerical workers; the wear and tear on the joints of neck and shoulders and back of farm labourers; the leg circulatory problems of those who stand for long periods of time with little

movement; the aural problems of those working in conditions of extreme noise.

Problems arising in this area include structural damage to organs and tissues, and local or general retardation of the movement of Qi and Xue in the Jing Luo.

(ii) Mental - Emotional

The majority of individuals suffer, to a greater or lesser degree, from dissatisfaction with their occupation; from boredom, apathy, frustration, depression or general stress. Retirement, and loss or lack of a job, can give rise to similar emotions. The Different types of emotional disharmony are discussed in Chapter 15.

Overwork

Overwork may result from one or more of the following: insecurity, greed, peer group pressure, perfectionism, ambition - whether for money, power or fame or the desire to further a political, religious or charitable cause - and so on. Also, a particular loss, or a generally unhappy life, may result in individuals immersing themselves in work, as others immerse themselves in alcohol.

Work is basically activity, and therefore excessive work will tend to deplete Yang. Work tends to injure Shen Qi, and also Shen Yang, and hence Pi Yang. Too much mental work and study are said to injure Pi. Also, the strain of too much exertion may damage Xin Yang.

If work is associated with mental and emotional stress, this may deplete Yin, with Deficient Yin of Shen, Gan and Xin; and perhaps Blazing Fire in Gan and Xin. This is especially likely in persons already tending to Deficient Yin.

Exercise

Exercise may be considered in three main categories:-

(i) Insufficient Exercise

Most people, and certainly most patients, in the West, take insufficient exercise, and this is a powerful contributing factor to disease. If circulation of Qi and Xue is sluggish, then the operation of all body systems will also be sluggish, resulting not only in diseases associated with stagnation of Qi and Xue, but also with those associated with Qi and Xue Deficiency and with the entry of External Factors due to Deficiency of Wei Qi.

(ii) Excessive Exercise

While a 1 mile jog might be scarcely enough for a lazy overweight 25-year-old with an undemanding job, it might be excessive for a 70-year-old with a heavy work load. Excessive exercise will have the same effect as too much physical work, it will weaken Qi of Shen and Xin.

(iii) Incorrect Exercise

As with nutrition, requirements of both type and amount of exercise vary with the individual, and individual requirements change with time. Commonsense and moderation are the key words here; a vigorous game of squash may be detrimental in a case of angina, just as parachuting is unwise for overweight patients with weak ankles. Less vigorous and drastic forms of exercise may be more appropriate here, such as swimming or hiking.

Exercise that is unsuitable for a particular patient is likely to lead to strain and injury of organs and tissues, and to disturbance of the healthy circulation of Qi and Xue.

Relationships

Diseases arising within the Body in situations of difficult relationships with other individuals are often patterns associated with emotional disharmony. The various types of emotional imbalance are discussed in Chapter 15.

Problems associated with close relationships may be especially difficult to help. This is due to the great amount of time that the individual has been, and is, exposed to close relations, and hence to the depth to which patterns of behaviour are ingrained, and to the power of the emotional pressures behind them.

Sex

Sex is a matter so closely interwoven with personal relationships as to be virtually inseparable from them. Hence, sexual problems are rarely of purely physical origin. For example, impotence, the inability to get or maintain an erection, is usually due to a combination of various emotional and mental factors, e.g. anxiety, guilt, lack of confidence, and is often in terms of a particular relationship.

Chinese texts generally regard excess sex as conducive to ill-health. This is discussed on pages 71-72.

With a population in excess of 1 billion, the Chinese do not emphasise problems arising from insufficient sex; although, as in any other area of health, both excess and deficiency may lead to difficulty, depending on the individual and the particular situation.

Trauma, Parasites and Pestilences

According to TCM, injury is accompanied by areas of local stagnation of Qi and Xue. Even after the local injury has healed, and the local signs of injury have disappeared, a site of potential weakness often remains that may be activated at a later date. Later recurrence of a problem in the area may occur when the flow of Qi and Xue has been weakened by age, cold, malnutrition, exhaustion, or further injury.

Obviously, an event such as the loss of a relative, is a shock to the emotional system, and also a physical trauma, such as the loss of a leg, also carries with it a component of emotional shock. What is not so apparent is that mental/emotional factors may contribute to or cause perhaps the majority of physical 'accidents' in the first place. So many car accidents, for example, are caused by tiredness, inattention, or the influence of alcohol or drugs. Tiredness may result from insomnia, so often due to emotional causes; inattention may be caused by depression, anger, or the escapism of day- dreaming; and consumption of alcohol and drugs results from emotional discontent.

Trauma includes all accidents and injuries, whether they involve other human beings, animals, plants or inanimate objects. Trauma includes, for example, burns, bites and stings. Parasites is a vague, general term, that includes infections and infestations. However, there is the further concept of Li Qi, or Pestilences, which are considered as External Disease Factors, but as more or less distinct from the Six Climatic Factors, and as able to invade even a healthy individual.

Treatment as a Disease Factor

Physical injury may follow incorrect acupuncture treatment or mistakes or difficulties during surgery. These injuries tend to lead to structural damage of the tissues, and either to obstruction of Qi and Xue, accompanied by dull or severe local pain, or to sites of chronic inflammation and irritation with redness, soreness and swelling. The former is often associated with local accumulation of Cold and Damp, and the latter with local accumulation of Damp and Heat.

The use of inappropriate type or dose of Western medicines may lead to illness. This also applies to herbal medicines, but to a lesser degree. Even correct use of a very large number of Western medicines may lead to illness through their side-effects upon the Body. This rarely occurs following correct use of herbal medicine.

The incorrect use, or the side-effects of the correct use, of Western medicines and treatments may result in deep and lasting disharmonies of the mind, the emotions, and the physical body. The signs of these drug-induced disharmonies are very common in the West, and can greatly confuse diagnosis. The practitioner must be aware of treatment as a common disease factor, and must assess this possibility in every case.

Secondary Factors

There are certain secondary Disease Factors, which may arise from the action of one or more of the primary Disease Factors which have been discussed above. Three of these Secondary Factors are extremely important in Chinese medicine, and are discussed in detail in later Chapters.

Stagnation	discussed on p. 180
Phlegm	discussed on p. 84
Internal Wind	discussed on p. 113

The Disease Factors are discussed at greater length in Chapter 17, in the section on Patient Education.

Summary

In ancient China, in Third World countries today, or indeed in any poor and mainly rural society, the External Factors of disease are predominant. Malnutrition and prolonged exposure to extremes of climate are major factors.

In the richer countries with greater industrial development, the pattern of illness is different. The Internal Factors, especially emotional and mental stress and disharmony, are the main factors originating, aggravating and perpetuating disease.

However, human societies and the ecosystem of this planet are in a process of constant change and development. The rate of change is accelerating with the growth of communications systems and of world population. In 50 years, the patterns of disease in all societies are likely to undergo great change, and the patterns of treatment must alter to match this.

Chapter

5

Patterns of Disease

Terminology
In Western medical terminology the word syndrome generally indicates a
commonly occurring combination of signs and symptoms, not necessarily always
due to the same cause. Hence, syndrome plus cause equals Disease.

Since this conception is alien to Chinese medical thought, the word syndrome is
avoided in this text and the phrase Pattern of Disharmony, or simply Disharmony,
is used to indicate any disharmonious pattern of Substances, Jing Luo, Zang Fu,
or Body generally. The word 'disease' is only used to mean a Pattern of
Disharmony, not a syndrome as in the Western sense. The word 'cause' has been
avoided, since it implies cause and effect. The phrase Disease Factor is used to
indicate an aspect of the overall pattern of Body and environment associated with
the origin or precipitation of imbalance. The origins of a Pattern of Disharmony
are seen in terms of an interacting combination of Disease Factors, not in terms of
a single cause. The word 'sign' is used in this book to mean both signs, the
objective indications of disease observed by the practitioner, and symptoms, the
subjective indications reported by the patient.

Classification of Patterns of Disease
A patient coming for diagnosis manifests various signs of disharmony. The
practitioner attempts to arrange these signs into a recognisable pattern, according
to the concepts of TCM.

The patient's signs are classified in terms of six main categories of disharmony:-

Yin Yang	Substances
Eight Principles	Jing Luo
Disease Factors	Zang Fu

The Patterns of Disharmony of the Substances and of the Disease Factors have already been discussed, those of the Jing Luo are covered by most major texts, and those of the Zang Fu are considered in later chapters of this book.

In Chinese medicine, the first stage of differential diagnosis is to classify the patient's signs in terms of the Patterns of Disharmony of the Eight Principles.

Patterns of Disharmony of the Eight Principles

The Eight Principles are four pairs of polar opposites:-

Table 5.1 Patterns of Disharmony of the Eight Principles

Yin	Yang
Interior	Exterior
Cold	Heat
Deficiency	Excess

Yin Yang is the basis of Chinese medicine; all physiology and pathology is founded on the principle of Yin Yang. The Eight Principles for the classification of Patterns of Disharmony are Yin Yang and three subdivisions of Yin Yang:- Cold and Heat, Deficiency and Excess, Internal and External. These three subdivisions extend the applications of Yin Yang in clinical practice.

Interior and Exterior
These two principles relate to the depth of the disease, and also to the direction of development of the disease. External diseases relate to the surface layers of the Body, and tend to move inward into the Body. Internal diseases relate to the interior of the Body, and may originate at these deeper levels.

Exterior patterns are generally associated with the invasion of the Body by one or more of the External Disease Factors. Such patterns are generally acute, of sudden onset and short duration, with such signs as aversion to wind and cold, fever and chills, headache, nasal congestion, sore or itchy throat, and superficial pulse.

Interior patterns may arise from eventual penetration by External Disease Factors from the superficial layers to the Interior of the Body; from direct invasion of Zang Fu by External Factors; or from internal Disharmonies of the Zang Fu.

Interior patterns are generally more serious and chronic, and of longer duration and more gradual onset. If there is fever it is generally high, with no fear of cold or wind. There may be vomiting, and changes in urine and stool, deeper pulse, and changes in the body of the tongue in addition to changes in tongue coat.

Cold and Heat
Patterns of Cold may be associated with invasion of the Body by such External Disease Factors as Cold, Wind and Damp; or they may relate to Internal patterns such as Deficient Yang or Deficient Qi of the Body in general, or of certain organ systems in particular.

Patterns of Heat may accompany invasion of the Body by such External Factors as Heat, Summer Heat, Wind, Dryness and Damp; or arise by transformation in the Body of such External Factors as Wind and Cold; or relate to Internal patterns such as Deficient Yin, or Damp Heat.

Cold patterns have signs such as cold limbs, aversion to cold, white face, clear copious secretions and urine, watery stool, lack of thirst, slow movement and slow tight pulse, and pale tongue with white coat. Discomfort is generally increased by cold and reduced by warmth.

Signs of Heat are generally the opposite of signs of Cold:- there is hot red skin, aversion to heat, reduced secretions and urine, constipation, thirst, excitability, rapid movement and rapid pulse, and red tongue with yellow coat. Discomfort is generally increased by heat and reduced by cold.

Deficiency and Excess

Deficiency generally refers to chronic Internal patterns associated with Deficiency of one or more of the Substances, and of one or more of the Zang Fu. Hence Deficiency patterns will have an underlying weakness and emptiness regardless of whether the Deficiency is predominantly of Yin or of Yang. In Deficiency, the antipathogenic factors are generally weak, and the pathogenic factors well-established in the Body.

Excess may refer to invasion of the Body by External Disease Factors, when the struggle between the pathogenic and antipathogenic factors is strong because the antipathogenic factors are not yet impaired. Excess may also refer to overactivity of one or more Zang Fu; or it may refer to local obstruction with associated local accumulation of Qi, Xue or Jin Ye.

Overall Deficiency is more likely to be chronic, with weakness and tiredness or inconsistent energy, weak or inconsistent voice, breathing and movements, weak, empty pulse, and tongue with little or no coat. Overall Excess is more likely to be acute, with heavy forceful voice, breathing and movements, discomfort aggravated by pressure, strong, full pulse and tongue with thick coat.

The main signs of Interior, Exterior, Cold, Heat, Deficiency and Excess are summarized in Table 5.2.

Yin and Yang

In TCM, Yin and Yang are the basis of physiology, pathology and differential diagnosis. All is seen in terms of the fundamental disharmony of Yin and Yang. A few examples of the signs of disharmony of Yin and of Yang are summarized in Table 5.3.

The Yin Pattern of Disharmony can be subdivided into the patterns of Cold, Deficiency and Interior; and the Yang Patterns of Disharmony can be subdivided into the patterns of Heat, Excess and Exterior; as shown in Table 5.1.

Combinations of the patterns of Yin or Yang with the patterns of the other Eight Principles, or with each other, are discussed later in this chapter.

Combinations of the Patterns of the Eight Principles

The dichotomy of Yin Yang, consisting of only two categories, Yin and Yang, is too limited to classify the patterns of disharmonies found in clinical practice, and is expanded into the Eight Principles. Indeed, Eight categories would also be too few, but this is extended by using combinations of the patterns of the Eight Principles.

Table 5.2 Main Signs of Interior, Exterior, Cold, Heat, Deficiency and Excess

Pattern	Signs	Pulse	Tongue
Interior	often chronic, with more gradual onset and longer duration, and more changes in urine and stool; fever,if present may be severe, with no aversion to cold	deep	changes in tongue body and coat
Exterior	often acute, with more sudden onset and shorter duration, and less changes in urine and stool; fever and chills, with aversion to wind cold or heat	superficial	changes in tongue coat
Cold	aversion to cold, cold limbs, white face, slow movement, quiet behaviour, no thirst, no perspiration, copious, clear urine, diarrhoea	slow tight	white coat ±pale body
Heat	aversion to heat, hot red skin, rapid movement, excitability, thirst, perspiration, dark urine, constipation	rapid	yellow coat ±red body
Deficiency	often chronic, with tiredness and weak voice, breathing and movements; discomfort often relieved by pressure	empty	little or no coat
Excess	often acute, with loud coarse voice, heavy breathing and movements; discomfort often aggravated by pressure	full	thick coat

Table 5.3 Signs of Disharmony of Yin and of Yang

Type of Sign	Yin	Yang
general	pale face, feels cold, aversion to cold, discomfort relieved by warmth and by pressure, no thirst or preference for warm drinks	red face, feels hot aversion to heat and pressure thirst and preferences for cool drinks
energy	tired, weak	forceful, restless
behaviour	underactive, quiet, withdrawn	overactive, noisy, outgoing
breathing and voice	weak shallow breathing, weak voice	deep heavy breathing, loud coarse voice
digestion	reduced appetite, abdominal distension	increased appetite, burning pain in epigastrium
excretion	copious clear urine, diarrhoea	scanty dark urine, constipation
reproduction	sexually underactive, scanty pale menses, white leucorrhoea	sexually overactive, profuse red menses, yellow leucorrhoea
pulse	deep, slow, empty	superficial, rapid, full
tongue	pale body; moist, thin white coat	red body; dry, thick yellow coat

However, by convention, not all possible combinations are used. For example, Excess Heat, Excess Cold, Deficient Heat, Deficient Cold, External Heat, External Cold, Internal Heat, Internal Cold, Deficient Yin and Deficient Yang, are commonly used categories; whereas External Yin, Internal Yin, External Yang, Internal Yang, External Excess, etc., are not.

48

Exterior and Heat, Interior and Heat; Exterior and Cold, Interior and Cold
These combinations patterns, more usually known as External Heat, Internal Heat, External Cold and Internal Cold respectively, have already been discussed in Chapter 4. They indicate whether the Disease Factors of Heat and Cold are predominantly of External or Internal origin. In these four combinations, the classification according to Disease Factors overlaps with the classification according to the Eight Principles, since the categories of Heat and Cold occur in both classifications.

The signs of the four combined patterns are summarized in Table 5.4:-

Table 5.4 Comparison of the Signs of Internal and External Cold, and Internal and External Heat

External Cold	Internal Cold
chills and fever	no fever
acute	chronic
superficial tight pulse	deep tight pulse
thin white tongue coat	thick white tongue coat

External Heat	Internal Heat
fever acute, with fear of wind	fever higher or more chronic, without fear of wind
superficial rapid pulse	full rapid pulse
red tongue with thin yellow coat	redder tongue with thicker yellower coat

These combined patterns are composed of the signs of one of the contributing patterns plus the signs of the other contributing pattern. For example, the pattern of External Heat is composed of Exterior signs, such as superficial pulse and thin tongue coat, plus Heat signs such as rapid pulse and yellow tongue coat. The pattern of External Cold also has Exterior signs, but in combination with signs of Cold, such as tight pulse and white tongue coat.

Excess and Heat, Deficiency and Heat, Excess and Cold, Deficiency and Cold
An individual in perfect harmony, with Yin and Yang in balance, and with no deficiencies of the Substances, can be summarized diagramatically as in Figure 5.1a:

Figure 5.1

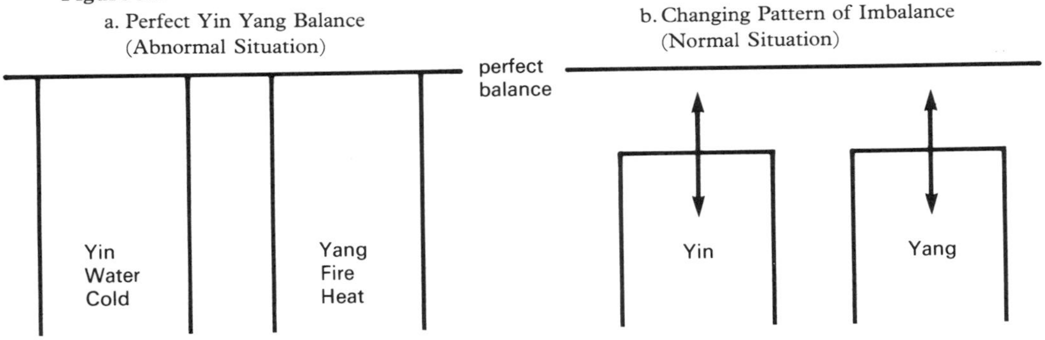

a. Perfect Yin Yang Balance (Abnormal Situation)

b. Changing Pattern of Imbalance (Normal Situation)

perfect balance

Yin Water Cold   Yang Fire Heat

Yin   Yang

In Figure 5.1, Yin and Yang, Water and Fire, Cold and Heat are in perfect balance. This is **not** the normal situation. In the normal or usual situation, Yin and Yang are not in perfect balance, and also one or more of the Substances is Deficient.

The normal human condition is of a greater or lesser degree of depletion and imbalance. As shown in Figure 5.1b, both Yin and Yang are usually Deficient, and their relative levels are continually changing.

If Qi is Deficient, then both Yin and Yang will also be Deficient, with a tendency to relatively greater Deficiency of Yang. If Xue is Deficient, both Yin and Yang will also be Deficient, with a tendency to relatively greater Deficiency of Yin. These relationships are summarized in Figure 5.2:-

Figure 5.2 Yin Yang Balance and Deficiencies of Qi and Xue

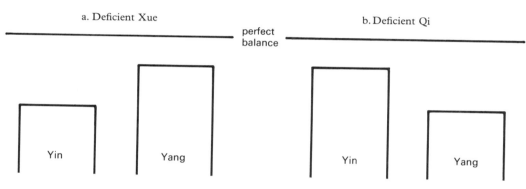

Yin and Yang are not only opposite but sustain and complement each other, so that, for example, a relative Deficiency of Yin may eventually lead to a Deficiency of both Yin and Yang, although the Deficiency of Yin remains relatively greater. Similarly, a relative Deficiency of Yang may eventually lead to a Deficiency of both Yin and Yang, with the emphasis on Deficient Yang.

This principle is often reflected in treatment. For example, in a case of Deficient Shen Yang, it is often not enough to strengthen Shen Yang; it is also necessary to strengthen Shen Yin to some degree, although the main emphasis of the treatment is on Shen Yang. The analogy here is of an oil lamp(3); the oil is the Yin, the flame is the Yang. If only the Yang, the flame, is increased, the lamp will only burn a short time. It is also necessary to increase the oil, the Yin, so that the lamp may burn longer.

Excess and Heat (Excess Yang), Deficiency and Heat (Deficient Yin)
These two patterns are also known as Excess Heat and Deficient Heat.

Excess Heat (Excess Yang)
In the pattern of Excess Heat shown in Figure 5.3a, Heat and Yang are in actual Excess. After a time, this Heat will damage the Yin and fluids of the Body, resulting in the pattern shown in Figure 5.3b.

Excess Heat is a combination of the patterns of Excess and Heat; and therefore has signs of Excess such as full pulse and thick tongue coat, along with signs of

Figure 5.3 Yin Yang Balance and Excess Heat (Excess Yang)

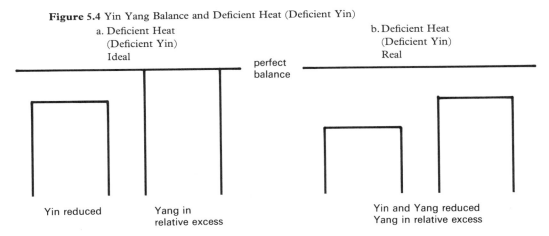

a. Excess Heat
(Excess Yang)

b. Prolonged Excess Heat
(Prolonged Excess Yang)

perfect
balance

Yin   Yang   Yin   Yang

Yin normal   Yang in real   Yin reduced   Yang in real
                  excess   excess

Heat such as rapid pulse and yellow tongue coat. Signs of this combined pattern are outlined in Table 5.5.

This is a pure Yang pattern, since both the contributing patterns of Excess and Heat are in themselves Yang. The two patterns complement each other and the signs are full, strong and forceful.

Deficient Heat (Deficient Yin)

The pattern of Deficient Heat or Deficient Yin is usually represented in textbooks as in Figure 5.4a. Here Yang is shown as normal, but in relative Excess over Yin which is Deficient. However, Defecient Yin is generally a pattern of chronic Deficiency, so that it will involve Deficiency of both Yin and Yang. This more realistic representation is shown in Figure 5.4b, where both Yin and Yang are shown as Deficient, but Yin is relatively more Deficient and Yang is relatively Excess.

Figure 5.4 Yin Yang Balance and Deficient Heat (Deficient Yin)

a. Deficient Heat
(Deficient Yin)
Ideal

b. Deficient Heat
(Deficient Yin)
Real

perfect
balance

Yin reduced   Yang in   Yin and Yang reduced
                   relative excess   Yang in relative excess

This pattern is a combination of the patterns of Deficiency and of Heat, with signs of Deficiency such as thin pulse and tongue with little or no coat, and of Heat such as rapid pulse with red tongue (see Table 5.5).

This is a mixed pattern, since one of the contributing patterns is Yin and the other Yang. The Yin signs of Deficiency modify the Yang signs of Heat, so that only the cheeks are red in contrast to the pattern of Excess Heat in which all the face is red.

Deficient Heat (Deficient Yin) is usually a chronic pattern associated with Internal Disease Factors; whereas Excess Heat is often an acute pattern associated wtih External Disease Factors.

The pattern of Deficient Heat is commonly known as Deficient Yin, since there is said to be insufficient Yin to control the Yang, or insufficient Water to control the Fire. Hence, there are signs of Heat, but with underlying weakness. For example, the patient may be restless, excited and talkative, with insomnia and irritability, as in Excess Heat. However, with Deficient Heat the signs are not so forceful, and are liable to alternate with signs of tiredness and exhaustion. Excess Heat is often associated with acute high fevers, and Deficient Heat is often associated with chronic Zang Fu disharmonies, especially Deficient Shen Yin.

Excess and Cold (Excess Yin), Deficiency and Cold (Deficient Yang)
These two patterns are alternatively known as Excess Cold and Deficient Cold.

Excess Cold (Excess Yin)
In the pattern of Excess Cold, shown in Figure 5.5a, Cold and Yin are in actual Excess. Eventually, this Excess of Cold will injure the Yang, resulting in the pattern shown in Figure 5.5b.

Figure 5.5 Yin Yang Balance and Excess Cold (Excess Yin)

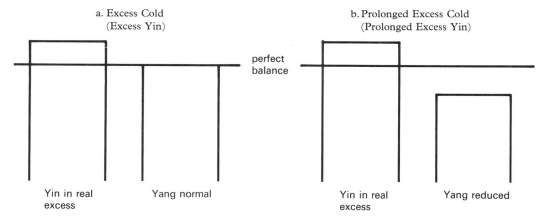

a. Excess Cold
(Excess Yin)

b. Prolonged Excess Cold
(Prolonged Excess Yin)

perfect
balance

Yin in real
excess

Yang normal

Yin in real
excess

Yang reduced

Excess Cold (Excess Yin) is a combination of the patterns of Excess, which is Yang, and of Cold, which is Yin. There are some signs of Excess, such as full pulse and thick tongue coat, and signs of Cold such as deep pulse and white tongue coat. The Yin aspect and the Yang aspect modify each other. This is in contrast to the pattern of Excess Heat, where both contributing patterns are Yang and complement each other. For example, in Excess Heat, the movements of the pulse and the body are strong and fast, whereas in Excess Cold they are strong but slow (see Table 5.5).

Deficient Cold (Deficient Yang)

The pattern of Deficient Cold or Deficient Yang is usually represented in textbooks as in Figure 5.6a. Here, Yin is shown as normal, but in relative Excess over Yang, which is Deficient. However, Deficient Yang is generally a pattern of chronic Deficiency, and this will eventually involve Deficiency of both Yin and Yang. The pattern is more realistically represented in Figure 5.6b, in which both Yang and Yin are shown as Deficient, but Yang is relatively more Deficient, and Yin is in relative Excess.

Figure 5.6 Yin Yang Balance and Deficient Cold (Deficient Yang)

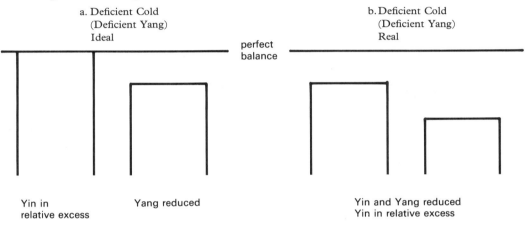

a. Deficient Cold
(Deficient Yang)
Ideal

b. Deficient Cold
(Deficient Yang)
Real

perfect balance

Yin in
relative excess   Yang reduced

Yin and Yang reduced
Yin in relative excess

Deficient Cold is a combination of the Yin pattern of Deficiency and the Yin pattern of Cold, so that it is a pure Yin pattern, just as Excess Heat is a pattern of pure Yang.

Both Cold and Deficiency are Yin, and both tend to lead to slowness and weakness of the circulation of Qi and Xue, so that both contribute to signs such as the pale tongue, and the slow weak movements of pulse and Body.

The pattern of Excess Cold tends to be more of External origin, whereas Deficient Cold tends to be more of Internal origin, although both Internal and External Disease factors may contribute to both patterns (see pages 32–33).

Deficient Cold is commonly known as Deficient Yang, since there is said to be insufficient Yang Heat to balance the Yin Cold. Also, since there is insufficient Yang to warm, move and retain the Water, there may be local accumulation of Damp or copious clear urination. In the pattern of Deficient Yang, there are signs of emptiness and weakness, in contrast to the signs of fullness and forcefulness that accompany Excess Cold.

In the patterns of Deficient Yin and Deficient Yang, the Excess of Yin or Yang is only relative or apparent; whereas in the patterns of Excess Cold and Excess Heat, the Excess of Yin(Cold) or Yang(Heat) are **actual** or real.

On page 23, the patterns of Deficient Yin and Deficient Yang are compared and contrasted with each other, and with the patterns of Deficient Qi and Deficient Xue.

Table 5.5 Comparison of the Signs of Excess and Deficient Cold, and Excess and Deficient Heat

Excess Cold (Excess Yin)	Deficient Cold (Deficient Yang)	Deficent Heat (Deficient Yin)	Excess Heat (Excess Yang)
cold limbs, aversion to cold, discomfort relieved by warmth aggravated by pressure	cold limbs, aversion to cold, discomfort relieved by warmth and by pressure	afternoon fever, malar flush, feverish sensation in palms and soles	high fever, whole body red and hot, discomfort relieved by cold, aggravated pressure
forceful slow movements	weak slow movements, lassitude, hypersomnia	weak rapid movements, restlessness, insomnia	forceful rapid movements, restlessness, delirium
no perspiration	daytime perspiration	night-time perspiration	perspiration
clear copious urination	clear copious urination	dark scanty urination	dark scanty urination
watery stools	watery stools	constipation	constipation
deep, slow, full pulse	slow, empty pulse	rapid, thin pulse	rapid, full pulse
pale tongue, thick white coat	pale tongue, thick white coat	red tongue, little or no coat	dark red tongue, thick yellow coat

Collapse of Yin or Yang

Under extreme conditions, Deficient Yin can become the pattern termed Collapse of Yin (Vanquished Yin) and Deficient Yang can become Collapse of Yang (Vanquished Yang). The signs of these extreme patterns are summarized in Table 5.6.

Table 5.6 Collapse of Yin and Collapse of Yang

Collapse of Yin	Collapse of Yang
flushed face; skin, hands and feet hot, aversion to heat; restlessness; thirst and preference for cold drinks; sticky perspiration; rapid respiration	pale face; skin and limbs cold, aversion to cold; listlessness; preference for warm drinks, profuse cold perspiration; feeble respiration
pulse flooding or thin and fast	pulse very minute, without strength
tongue red and dry with little or no coat	tongue pale and moist

Collapse of Yin may arise from extreme loss of Jin Ye, as in excessive perspiration, vomiting or haemorrhage. This is an emergency situation, where the Yin must be restored, and where the patient may be near collapse, as in Heat stroke.

Collapse of Yang relates to total exhaustion, and again needs emergency treatment, and often occurs just before shock. Collapse of Yin or Yang is more extreme than Deficiency of Yin or Yang, and can injure the Body more severely. Collapse of Yin and Collapse of Yang can quickly transform into each other, and when both Yin and Yang are in Collapse, the patient may be near to death.

True Heat and Illusionary Cold: True Cold and Illusionary Heat

These two patterns are also extreme forms of Yin Yang imbalance. The pattern of True Heat and Illusionary Cold may arise during a disease of extreme Heat. There may be signs of excessive Heat such as great thirst, delirium, full rapid pulse and dry tongue with yellow coat; then suddenly the limbs may go cold whilst the other signs remain unaltered. This is said to correspond to the Yin and fluids being greatly depleted, and are suddenly being pushed to the extremities by the excessive Fire and Yang. The Heat is therefore said to be True, and the Cold to be Illusionary.

True Cold and Illusionary Heat may arise during an illness of excessive Cold, with cold limbs and minute pulse. Then suddenly the patient may be agitated, as if in a Heat disharmony. This is said to be due to the Yin and fluid being so great, and the Yang and Fire so small, that the Yang floats to the surface of the Body, where it is temporarily given the appearance of Heat. The Cold is therefore said to be True, and the Heat to be Illusionary.

Apparent Contradictions

The pattern of signs manifested by a patient in the clinic can often seem complex, confusing and contradictory. Signs of Heat may be mixed with signs of Cold, there may be signs of both Deficient Yin and Deficient Yang, and signs of Interior and of Deficiency may co-exist with signs of Exterior and of Excess.

Internal and External

As discussed in Chapter 4, both Internal and External causes may contribute to a Pattern of Disharmony; as in the case of Internal and External Cold interacting with Deficient Shen Yang (Figure 4.1), Internal and External Heat interacting with Deficient Shen Yin (Figure 4.2), and Internal and External Damp interacting with Deficient Pi Qi (Figure 4.3).

As External Factors invade the Body, they may change their nature, e.g. Cold Wind may become Heat subsequent to invasion; and they may progress deeper into the Body and become termed Internal rather than External, or as well as External. These changes are described in the Classification of the Six Stages (Diseases due to Cold), and the Classifications of Wei Qi Yin Xue and of San Jiao (Diseases due to Heat). Discussion of these three major classifications is outside the scope of this book.

Deficiency and Excess

A patient may have signs of overall Deficiency of Qi and Xue. In addition, they may have signs of local Excess due to local stagnation and accumulation of Qi, Xue or Jin Ye, in a particular area of the Body, perhaps due to trauma or local invasion of Cold and Damp.

Also, there may be apparent signs of Excess with genuine underlying Deficiency, as in the pattern of Deficient Yin (Deficient Heat). Alternatively there may be patterns of Excess in one Zang Fu, existing simultaneously with patterns of Deficiency in other Zang Fu. For example, there may be Deficiency of Pi leading to production of Phlegm, linked with the Excess pattern of Retention of Phlegm in Fei.

Besides being woven together, patterns of Excess and Deficiency may transform into one another. For example, chronic asthma of the Deficient type, i.e. involving Deficient Qi of Shen and Fei, predisposes the Body to invasion by External Cold. Such invasion may lead to an acute attack of asthma of the Excess type. This temporary Excess pattern usually later subsides into asthma of the Deficiency type. Hence, there is a recurring pattern of underlying chronic Internal Deficiency, with periodic acute crises of the External Excess type.

Cold and Heat, Yin and Yang

The simultaneous occurrence of signs of Deficient Yin and Deficient Yang is discussed in Chapter 3, on page 22, and in Case History 7 on page 244.

Qualification of the Classifications of the Eight Principles

So far, in this discussion, the signs of an individual's Pattern of Disharmony have been classified in terms of Yin Yang, the Eight Principles, and combinations of the patterns of the Eight Principles with each other.

However, this classification of Eight Principles is usually qualified in terms of the Patterns of Disharmony of other categories:-

Disease Factors   Substances   Jing Luo   Zang Fu

Examples of such qualification of the classification of the Eight Principles are given in Table 5.7.

Table 5.7 Qualification of the classification of the Eight Principles

Qualification	Examples
Disease Factors	Internal Damp, External Wind Cold
Substances	Deficient Jing, Heat in Xue
Jing Luo	Invasion of Gan Jing Luo by External Cold
Zang Fu	Deficient Shen Yin, Hyperactive Xin Fire

For example, there might be signs of an Internal disharmony in terms of the Eight Principles' classification:- chronic pattern, with gradual onset, changes in urine and stool, and thick tongue coat. However, using the categories of the Disease Factor, the classification of the patient's pattern in terms of the Eight Principles can be qualified or extended. Feelings of heaviness and fullness in head and chest, slippery pulse, and greasy tongue coat indicate the Pernicious Influence Damp. The classification of the patient's pattern now becomes Internal Damp.

Similarly, a pattern which is of Deficiency in terms of the Eight Principles:- patient weak, with thin pulse and thin tongue coat - may be qualified in terms of the Patterns of Disharmony of the Substances. For example, there may be premature baldness, loss of teeth and senility, indicating a disharmony of Jing. The overall classification of the patient's pattern is therefore Deficient Jing.

The patient may also be classified in terms of the patterns of other systems, for example the Six Divisions, Wei Qi Ying Xue, San Jiao, the Eight Extra Channels, the Five Phases, and the Ten Heavenly Stems and the Twelve Earthly Branches.

However, in clinical practice, the fundamental systems for the classification of the patients Patterns of Disharmony are:-

Yin Yang	Eight Principles	Disease Factors
Substances	Jing Luo	Zang Fu

Common Disease Patterns

Finally, TCM recognises various Common Disease Patterns, which may involve some or all of the five main categories of disharmony listed above. The Common Disease Patterns listed in some modern Chinese texts (9,13,18) are a curious mixture of presenting signs, Western syndromes or diseases, and Chinese disease patterns. For example:-

Table 5.8 Components of Common Disease Patterns

Component	Example
Presenting sign	insomnia, oedema, headache
Western syndrome or disease	malaria, arthritis, hyperthyroidism
Chinese Disease Pattern	Wei pattern, Bi pattern, Xiao Chuan

All three categories have been included under the phrase Common Disease Patterns, since they overlap, and often no clear distinction exists.

The confusion arises from the use of Western terms, with their specific Western medical connotations, as approximations for Chinese terms, which may have rather different meanings. For example, the Western term asthma is used as a translation for the Chinese pattern Xiao Chuan, but the two concepts are different, based on very different theories of health and disease. Also, some Western syndromes have no equivalent in TCM, for example cholecystitis and cholelithiasis. The signs of these Western syndromes are included in the Chinese patterns which approximate to jaundice, hypochondriac pain and some forms of gastric pain. Furthermore, one Western syndrome may include a variety of Chinese patterns, for example hyperthyroidism may include up to six different Chinese patterns. Alternatively, one Chinese pattern may cover a number of Western syndromes, for example Hyperactive Gan Fire is involved in some forms of essential hypertension, glaucoma, menorrhagia and emotional disturbances.

Summary

This chapter dealt with the classification of Patterns of Disharmony in Traditional Chinese Medicine. The Eight Principles' classification was discussed in some detail, since it is the initial stage of Differential Diagnosis, and since the diagnostic methods of tongue and pulse analysis are described in terms of the Eight Principles. Also the pathologies and Patterns of Disharmony of the Zang Fu are in terms of the Eight Principles, the Disease Factors and the Substances.

This ends Part I of this book. Part II is concerned with the Zang Fu, beginning with Chapter 6, which is a brief overview.

Part
2

Zang Fu

Chapter
6

Zang Fu

The Zang Fu form the central core of Traditional Chinese Medicine; physiology and pathology are in terms of the Zang Fu. The Zang Fu may be regarded as the organ systems of TCM, provided that it is understood that they do not so much refer to structures as to functional interrelationships, and that there is not necessarily a close correspondence between the Zang Fu and the organ system of Western medicine.

Origins of Confusion

Considerable confusion has arisen in the past on the topic of the Zang Fu, for five main reasons:-

1. Lack of sufficient accurate information on TCM.
2. Use of non-Chinese Asian material.
3. Over-emphasis and misapplication of Five Phase Theory.
4. Theoretical inventions of Western teachers.
5. Application of Western thinking and Western concepts to TCM.

   In the early days of the Western Colleges of Acupuncture, there was a serious lack of adequate, accurate information on the physiology and pathology of TCM. To compensate for this lack, material from Japan, Korea, Vietnam and elsewhere, was incorporated into course material and in some cases, was further supplemented by the home-grown theories of certain Western teachers. The resultant mixture of material was often inaccurate, inadequate and confusing, and, by definition, not Traditional Chinese Medicine.

A specific example of this was the gross over-use, and frequent misapplication, of the Theory of Five Phases, often mistranslated as The Theory of The Five Elements. This arose partly from severe lack of knowledge of the Eight Principles' Patterns and of Zang Fu physiology, and in certain cases colleges adopted the unfortunate position of teaching diagnosis and treatment largely or solely in terms of the Five Phase Theory. Since there is an excellent recent analysis of the importance of the Five Phase Theory by Kaptchuk and Bensky (12), it will not be considered further here.

In the last few years, especially with the publication of certain excellent texts (9,12,18) and with the availability of the 3 month preliminary and advanced acupuncture courses in Nanjing, and elsewhere in the People's Republic of China, sufficient accurate information on TCM has become available. Although the adoption of this material by the Western Colleges is a gradual, and in some cases, a slow process, it will eventually replace the confusing pastiche of non-Chinese material. Such concepts as the Theory of the Five Phases will then be seen in their proper context and perspective.

The greatest remaining problem will be the strong tendency to apply Western thought processes and Western concepts to TCM. Western thinking tends to be reductive and analytic, attempting to separate the parts of the phenomenon from each other, in order to study each part in isolation. Chinese thinking tends to be intuitive and synthetic, grouping phenomena together into patterns of functional interrelationships.

TCM is a complete and self-sufficient system of logic, which does not need the addition of concepts from other sources in order to function satisfactorily in both theory and practice. Indeed, the mixing of Chinese and Western concepts, or the misinterpretation and mistranslation of Chinese concepts, in terms of Western terminology, only leads to confusion. For example, The Western mind thinks of the liver as a solid, physical object, and views its function in terms of its biochemical, histological and anatomical structure. If the Chinese concept, Gan, is translated as liver, then the Western mind tends to see the Chinese organ system in these Western terms. However, Chinese medicine thinks less in terms of structures and more in terms of functional interrelationships; and also, the functions of Gan are not the same as those of the liver of Western medicine. TCM does not see the functions of Gan as storage of glycogen, iron, copper, and vitamin B12; nor as production of heparin and prothrombin. In TCM, the main function of Gan is promotion of the Free-flowing of Qi.

Furthermore, some Western organ systems, for example the various endocrine organs have no Chinese equivalent; and one Fu system, the San Jiao, is purely a concept of physiological relationships without an associated physical organ. Attempts to link specific endocrine glands to specific Zang Fu, or the San Jiao to a specific Western system, do not improve the clinical practice of TCM and usually produce further confusion.

In this book, the Chinese names of Zang Fu are used throughout, and the sooner the Chinese names are adopted in the West, and the use of Western terms in TCM abandoned, the sooner the Western confusion and misconception regarding Zang Fu will die down.

The Twelve Zang Fu

This book does not describe the Zang Fu in terms of either the organs of Western medicine, or of the Theory of Five Phases, but in terms of Yin Yang and the transformation and circulation of the Substances.

The function of the Zang Fu is to receive the air, food and drink from the external environment, and to transform these into the Substances and the waste products. The waste products are excreted, and the Substances circulated throughout the Body, and over the Body surface. Within the Body, Substances circulate both within and outside of the Jing Luo network, to supply all the systems and Tissues of the Body. The Zang Fu are also responsible for maintaining a harmonious interaction between the Body and the external environment.

The Six Zang, and their paired Fu, are listed in Table 6.1, along with the Chinese name, Western name, and Western abbreviation for each.

Zang and Fu

The Zang are relatively more Yin, solid, and internal, and are responsible for the formation, transformation, storage, release and regulation of the pure Substances:- Qi, Xue, Jing, Jin Ye, and Shen*.

The Fu are relatively more Yang, hollow, and external, and are responsible for the reception and storage of food and drink, and for the passage and absorption of their transformation products, and for the excretion of wastes.

Hence, the Fu are continually filling and emptying, filling with food and drink from the outside, or with digestion products, and emptying these products into the next Fu, or voiding the waste materials to the outside.

Table 6.1 Zang Fu

Zang			Fu		
Chinese words	English approximation	Abbrev-iation	Chinese words	English approximation	Abbrev-iation
Shen	Kidneys	KID	Pang Guang	Bladder	BL
Pi	Spleen	SP	Wei	Stomach	ST
Gan	Liver	LIV	Dan	Gall Bladder	GB
Xin	Heart	HE	Xiao Chang	Small Intestine	SI
Fei	Lungs	LU	Da Chang	Large Intestine	LI
Xin Bao	Pericardium	P	San Jiao	Triple Burner	TB

In contrast, the Zang do not communicate directly with the outside and transform the impure products from the Fu into pure substances which they store and release.

There are, of course, exceptions; Fei, although Zang, communicates directly with the external environment via respiration; Dan, although Fu, receives, stores and releases a pure substance, bile; and San Jiao is not associated with a physical organ, but can be regarded in terms of certain functional interrelationships of the other Zang Fu. Finally, Xin Bao is largely disregarded as a Zang system, its functions being included under Xin.

The Five Zang — Xin, Fei, Pi, Gan and Shen — are the heart of Chinese Medicine, and are more important than the six Fu organ systems. The perception of patterns of Disease of the five Zang systems, forms the central theme of diagnosis and treatment in TCM.

Zang Fu Pairs

Some of the pairings of Zang and Fu systems have considerable clinical relevance, while others do not. For example, there are very close links between Gan and Dan, Pi and Wei, and Shen and Pang Guang. However, the links between Xin and Xiao Chang, and Fei and Da Chang, are more tenuous and Patterns of Disharmony of Xiao Chang and Da Chang tend to be included in Patterns of Disharmony of Pi and Wei, and to be treated by points on the Pi and Wei channels. The links between Xin Bao and San Jiao are especially vague. Xin Bao is not generally regarded as separate from Xin, in the context of chronic disease; and the functions of Xin Bao, in the protection of Xin, and of San Jiao, in regulation of the Water Passages, are far apart.

Dan, Wei and Pang Guang have few Patterns of Disharmony separate from their respective Zang. Their physiology and pathology are mainly included in that of the dominant Zang system, though with emphasis more on the Yang, External aspects related to digestion and excretion. Whilst these three Fu have relatively little existence separate from their Zang organ system, their channels have a greater range of independent signs and symptoms, since the Pang Guang, Dan and Wei channels are the largest on the Body.

Summary

The Zang Fu are the core of TCM, just as they are at the centre of the organizational framework of the Body. To avoid confusion on this topic, it is essential to adhere to Chinese concepts and patterns of thinking, and not to mix these with concepts from any other system. For example, the Zang Fu of TCM are a completely different set of concepts from the organs of Western medicine, and should not be confused with them.

In this chapter, the functions of the Zang Fu were mentioned, and Zang and Fu compared. It was pointed out that some of the customary pairings of Zang and Fu may have been made more from reasons of theoretical neatness, than from genuine clinical observations.

In Chapters 7 to 11, each chapter discusses the functions, Origins of Disharmony, and Patterns of Disharmony of a Zang system, with a separate section on its paired Fu. Chapter 12 deals briefly with Xin Bao, and then in some detail with the difficult concept of San Jiao. Chapter 13 reviews the Zang Fu in terms of functions and Patterns of Disharmony.

Chapter
7

Shen (Kidneys) and Pang Guang (Bladder)

Shen

Functions

1. Stores Jing
   a. Rules birth, growth, development, and reproduction
   b. Rules bones
2. Foundation of Yin Yang
3. Rules the Water
4. Rules Reception of Qi
5. Opens into the Ears; Manifests in the Hair

This study of the Zang Fu starts with Shen, since Shen is the Root of Life, the Root of Qi, the Foundation of Yin and Yang, and the Foundation of the Water and Fire within the Body.

Stores Jing
Prenatal Jing from the parents is the origin of the Body, hence Shen is called the Root of Life. Since Prenatal Qi is the basis of Postnatal Qi, Shen is the Root of Qi.

Prenatal Jing comes before everything in the Body, even before the division into Yin Yang. Hence, Shen is the origin and the Foundation of Yin Yang, and of Water and Fire within the Body.

Prenatal Jing is considered irreplaceable; it can be conserved but not replaced. Postnatal Jing can be replenished from the energies from food and drink.

Areas of Confusion

Confusion arises for Western students due to the overlap of four closely related concepts:-

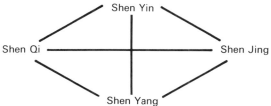

To clarify this confusion, the following four pairs of concepts are discussed below:-

Shen Qi and Shen Jing   Shen Jing and Shen Yang
Shen Qi and Shen Yang   Shen Jing and Shen Yin

Shen Qi and Shen Jing

The term Shen Qi can be used in the inclusive sense, to include Shen Jing along with all other activities of Shen; or it can be used in the more limited sense of Shen Qi as opposed to Shen Jing. Unfortunately, it is not always clear which sense predominates in the use of the phrase 'Shen Qi'. In clinical practice, there is considerable overlap between the two concepts, Deficient Shen Jing and Deficient Shen Qi, and in some cases they are used synonymously. However, Deficient Shen Jing relates more to problems of reproduction and development, whereas Deficient Shen Qi relates more to the Failure to Receive Qi, and to Deficient Shen Yang.

Shen Qi and Shen Yang.

Again, Shen Qi may be used in the inclusive sense, to include both Shen Yang and Shen Yin. However, especially in the clinic, it may be used in the more restricted sense, for example the pattern of Deficient Shen Qi, which tends to progress to the more severe pattern of Deficient Shen Yang, and not to the pattern of Deficient Shen Yin.

Shen Jing and Shen Yang : Shen Jing and Shen Yin

As stated on page 14, Shen Jing has its Yin and Yang functions, which overlap with the functions of Shen Yin and Shen Yang. However, Shen Yin and Shen Yang are more general categories, whereas Shen Jing (Yin) and Shen Jing (Yang) refer to the more specialised field of influence of Jing, i.e. reproduction, development, Bones, etc.

Shen Jing rules birth, growth, development, reproduction and the formation and function of Marrow, Bones, Brains and Xue. The Yin aspect of Jing provides the material base for the formation of Jing-related Tissues, for example Marrow, Bones, Brain, Xue and sperm, and also moistens and nourishes them. The Yang aspect of Jing is responsible for the warming, movement and activation of the Jing-related processes.

Functions of Jing

Jing circulates in the Jing Luo system, and in particular in the network of the Eight Extra Channels, to the Zang Fu and the Body, especially to the Curious Organs. Jing has a special link with the Curious Organs, since not only are all of them nourished and maintained by Jing, but for some of them, for example Marrow and Xue, Jing is involved in their formation.

The Jing circulating in the channel system becomes a part of the harmony of the Substances of the Body. For example, the Yang aspect of Jing may be involved with the Wei Qi in protecting the Body from External Invasion; and may be involved with Yuan Qi and Shen Yang in activating the formation, transformation and transportation of Qi, Xue and Jin Ye within the Body.

Rules the Bones

Marrow is formed from the Yin aspect of Shen Jing, and itself gives rise to the Brain, the Sea of Marrow, and to the Bone Marrow, which then gives rise to part of Xue.

Hence the proper formation and functioning of the Bones and Brain are dependent on the proper functioning of Shen, and on a sufficient supply of Jing. Shen is responsible for the fluidity of movement of the Body, and if Shen Jing is Deficient, there may be problems with the development and functioning of bones and joints, and therefore with movement.

Although, in TCM, the Zang associated with consciousness, mind and spirit is Xin, since it is the Residence of Shen*, the Brain was seen, at least by some authorities, to be involved in consciousness in a limited sense. The Brain is linked with the Orifices of the Senses, specifically those connected with eyes and ears, and if the Qi in the head is disorderly, the Orifices of the Senses are disrupted, so that the ears do not hear properly, the eyes do not see properly, and the person becomes dizzy and may lose consciousness.

Rules Birth, Growth, Development, Reproduction and Senescence

In its prenatal aspect, Jing is responsible for the transmission of inheritance; or, in Western terms, for the transmission of the genetic make-up of the parents, via sperm and ovum, to the offspring.

Shen links with the Uterus via Bao Mai, Ren Mai and Chong Mai, and is vital to the processes of conception, pregnancy and childbirth. Shen Jing is responsible for the formation of Yin Yang, and for the origin of Qi within the Body, and controls the cycles of further growth and differentiation. The 'Nei Jing' outlines the 7 year and 8 year cycles of growth and development in women and men respectively. These involve growth and development of bones and teeth, hair and reproductive system, sexual maturity and decline, and senescence.

Foundation of Yin Yang

Shen is the Foundation of Yin Yang, and of Fire and Water, both within the Body generally, and within the other Zang Fu. Shen Yang is the source of the Yang of all the Zang Fu, and Shen Yin is the source of all their Yin. Confusion arises due to the overlap of the following Concepts:-

Yang	Yin
Shen Yang	Shen Yin
Shen Fire	Shen Water
Shen Jing (Yang aspect)	Shen Jing (Yin aspect)
Ming Men Fire	
Yuan Qi	

Some authorities consider Ming Men, the Gate of Life, to be insubstantial, to be located between the Kidneys, and to be associated with the Fire of the Body. Other authorities associate Ming Men with the right Kidney, but in either case, Ming Men Fire, or Gate of Life Fire, is considered to be responsible for warming and activating the processes of the body. In clinical practice, the manifestation of Kidney Fire, Kidney Yang, Ming Men Fire and Yuan Qi are often regarded as more or less identical. The Yang aspect of Shen Jing may also be used synonmously with these, or may refer specifically to the reproductive functions.

Shen Rules the Water
Shen rules both the Fire of the Body, Ming Men Fire, and also the Water of the Body, Jin Ye. Shen is the Foundation of Fire and Water, and governs their balance within the Body.

The overlap of the concepts of Water and Jin Ye has been dealt with on page 15. Comparing the terms Water and Yin, Yin is a more inclusive concept than Water, which is but one aspect of Yin. Besides moistening and cooling, Yin also has the functions of nourishment and of providing a material base for formation of Structures.

The division into Yin and Yang includes the division into Fire and Water, which may manifest as Dryness and Damp, and hence as inflammation and oedema. Deficient Yang is associated with the Yin condition of the oedema. Excess Damp, accumulation of Fluids, and oedema. Deficient Yin is associated with the Yang condition of Excess Dryness and Heat, Deficient Jin Ye and inflammation.

A specific example of this is the special relationship between Shen and Fei in the movement of Jin Ye, as shown in Figure 7.1.

Deficient Shen Yin may result in Deficient Fei Yin, which may result in inflammation of Fei. Deficient Shen Yang and Qi, and Deficient Fei Yang, may result in deficient movement of Jin Ye, and hence in accumulation of fluid. Shen governs Jin Ye metabolism, and the cycle of fluid circulation within the Body, via its relationship with other Zang Fu. This is summarized in Figure 7.2 below.

Food and drink, received in Wei, are transformed by the action of Pi and Wei, especially the former, into purer and impurer fractions of Jin Ye. The denser fraction is passed from Wei to Xiao Chang, and thence to Pang Guang and Da Chang, for storage and excretion. Pi sends the purer, lighter, fraction as a vapour up to Fei, where a further separation takes place. The lightest fraction is dispersed by Fei to the skin, and the denser fraction is distributed by Fei throughout the Body. When the circulating fluids become impure, they are liquified and sent down by Fei to Shen. In Shen, this impure fraction is separated into denser and lighter components. The denser part is passed to Pang Guang for storage and excretion with possibly some transformation and reabsorption. The purer, lighter, part is vapourised by Shen and sent up to Fei, where it re-enters the fluid circulation cycle.

Figure 7.1 Shen, Fei and Jin Ye

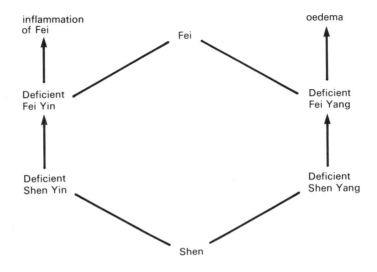

Figure 7.2 Cycle of Jin Ye Circulation

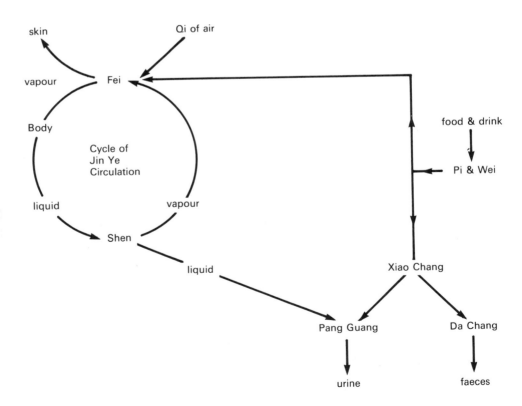

In this cycle, Shen Yang, alternatively termed Yuan Qi, or Ming Men Fire, is responsible for the Yang functions of warming, activating and moving, especially in three areas:-

1. Transformation and Transportation of food and drink by Pi and Wei.
2. Vapourisation of Jin Ye by Shen and their movement to Fei.
3. Processing of Jin Ye in Pang Guang.

Rules Reception of Qi
Fei is said to send Qi down to Shen, which receives it and holds it down. If either or both Fei or Shen are Deficient, and either Fei does not properly send down, or Shen does not properly hold down the Qi, the Qi in Fei becomes Rebellious. The Fei cannot properly perform its function of Dispersing and Descending Qi, and the inhalation process, which is dependent on Shen as well as Fei, becomes disrupted, causing shortness of breath, asthma, etc.

Opens into the Ears, and Manifests in the Hair
Although, as discussed on page 176, Shen is not the only Zang Fu concerned with the ears, nor are the ears the only sense organs influenced by Shen, the 'Nei Jing' states a special relationship between Shen and ears. Also, although Shen Jing is not the only factor affecting growth of head hair, see page 173, it is one of traditional importance.

Patterns of Disharmony

Deficient Shen Jing
Deficient Shen Yang
Deficient Shen Yin
Shen Fails to Receive Qi
Water Overflowing

The foundations of Shen pathology are the Deficiencies of Shen Qi, Shen Jing, Shen Yin and Shen Yang, and also the failure of Shen to Receive Qi, and to Govern Water.

Just as there is considerable overlap between the four pairs of concepts, Shen Qi, Shen Jing, Shen Yin and Shen Yang, there is similar overlap between the four Deficiency patterns, Deficient Shen Qi, Deficient Shen Jing, Deficient Shen Yin and Deficient Shen Yang. Here, the pattern Deficient Shen Jing is taken to include Deficient Shen Qi and Deficient Shen Jing, without bias to Yin or Yang. The pattern of Deficient Shen Yang indicates Deficiency of the Yang aspects of both Shen Qi and Shen Jing; similarly the pattern of Deficient Shen Yin refers to the Yin aspect of both Shen Qi and Shen Jing. The meaning given to each of these four patterns in any particular book can only be gained from a careful study of the signs listed under each pattern.

Origins of Shen Patterns of Disharmony
The origins of the Patterns of Disharmony of Shen are summarized in Figure 7.3 below.

Deficient Prenatal Jing

If the Jing of the parents is Deficient, then the Jing of the child may also be Deficient. If one or both of the parents are too old, exhausted or unhealthy, prior to conception, or the birth is premature, the Jing of the child may be Deficient.

Excess sex

What is excess sexual activity for one person, may not be excess for another; it depends on the state of health of a particular person, at a particular time. If a person is young with a strong constitution and good health, he is likely to be able to engage safely in more sexual activity than a person who is old and ill, with a weak constitution. However, not just the quantity but the quality of sexual activity is important. Sexual activity when a person is exhausted or emotionally upset, may not only aggravate these conditions but also deplete Jing.

Figure 7.3 Origins of Shen Disharmonies

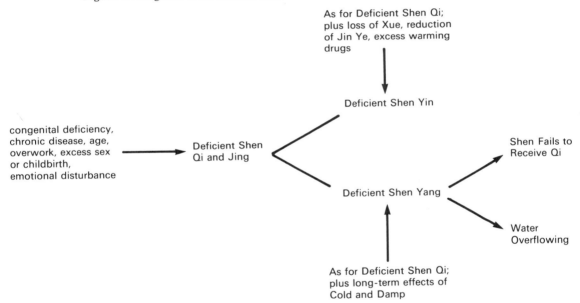

The 'Nei Jing' calls winter the time of Closing and Storing, when the energies of the Body go deeper, and when the Yang of the Body should not be disturbed; hence sexual activity should be reduced in this season. Spring, when the Yang of the Body rises and becomes active, is the time when sexual activity is naturally at its maximum.

Traditionally, Jing Deficiency due to excess sexual activity is greater in men than in women, although it occurs in both; and women suffer loss of Jing in childbirth, especially from a number of births following closely upon each other.

Excess sex depletes Jing, and may also deplete Shen Yang or Shen Yin. Which of these predominates, depends on whether the individual initially tends to Deficient Shen Yang or Deficient Shen Yin. If the initial tendency is to Deficient Shen Yin, then excess sexual activity will aggravate this condition by further depleting Jin Ye. For a person who tends to Deficient Shen Yang, excess sex will further deplete Ming Men Fire and Yang, thus aggravating this condition.

Emotional Disturbance
Severe acute fear or fright may damage Shen Yang with sudden loss of control over defecation and urination, the temporary loss of the capacity of Yang to hold things within the Body. Chronic fear can similarly cause enuresis by damage to Shen Yang, and is especially common in children. In individuals with initial tendency to Deficient Shen Yin, chronic fearful anxiety may damage Shen Yin, and signs of restlessness and insomnia may arise from subsequent Deficiency of Xin Yin, see page 130.

Other factors
Jing naturally decreases with age, but this process may be aggravated by chronic illness and overwork, since these two factors will cause Deficiency of other Zang Fu, such as Pi and Wei, resulting in poor replenishment of Post- natal Jing.

Deficient Shen Jing

Signs

Bones	late or incomplete fontanelle closure in infants, slow physical development, generally poor skeletal development, brittle bones, lumbar soreness, weakness of knees, poor teeth
Brain	slow mental development, mental dullness, poor memory, premature senility, dizziness
Ears	deafness, tinnitus
Reproduction	weak sexual activity, amenorrhoea, infertility, etc.
Hair	greying and premature hair loss
Pulse	deep, weak
Tongue	various

Pathology
This list of signs of Deficient Shen Jing assumes that Yin and Yang are equally Deficient, and that there are no signs of Heat or Cold. Generally, in practice, Yin and Yang are not equally Deficient and one or the other predominates. In this book, patterns which are predominantly of the Deficient Yang aspect of Jing are listed under Deficient Shen Yang and those of the Deficient Yin aspect of Jing are listed under Deficient Shen Yin. Some texts omit this category of Deficient Shen Jing (5), and deal only with the patterns of Deficient Shen Yang and Deficient Shen Yin, and their derivative categories.

Deficient Shen Jing signs include problems of birth, development, reproduction and ageing, with specific reference to formation and function of systems governed by Shen:- Bones, Brain, Ears and Hair. For example, Deficient Jing results in Deficient Marrow, and thus in weakness of Bones and Brain.

A deep weak pulse is often a sign of general Shen Deficiency, but the tongue pattern will vary according to whether the Deficiency is predominantly of Yin or of Yang.

Treatment

The principle of treatment is to strengthen Shen Jing, using reinforcing method, and using such points as:-

Taixi	KID.3	
Shenshu	BL.23	Strengthen Shen.
Guanyuan	Ren 4	
Zusanli	ST.36	Strengthens replenishment of Postnatal Jing.
Dazhui	BL.11	Meeting point of Bones, strengthens Bones.
Xuanzhong	GB.39	Meeting point of Marrow, strengthens Bones.

Various points may be added for specific problems, for example Yifeng, TB.17, for tinnitus, Yingu, KID.10, for problems of the knee joint, or Yaoyangguan, Du 3, for problems of the back.

Common Disease Patterns

Deficient Shen Jing may be a component of various disease patterns, including slow physical and mental development in children, infertility, tinnitus and premature senility.

Deficient Shen Yang

Signs

General Deficient Yang	bright, pale face, aversion to cold, cold limbs, lassitude, apathy
Deficient Jing (Yang)	sore cold back, weakness and cold in knees, reduced sexual drive, impotence, sterility, spermatorrhoea, loose teeth, deafness, etc.
Jin Ye	copious clear urine, incontinence, or reduced urine and oedema
Deficient Pi Yang	loss of appetite, loose stools, lassitude and debility
Pulse	deep, weak, slow
Tongue	pale flabby, perhaps with a thin white coat

Pathology

The functions of Yang are to move, warm and activate the Body processes, and to protect and hold in and hold up the Body components. Hence Deficient Yang results in Deficient warmth, and hence feelings of cold. The Deficient movement contributes to the lassitude and to the deep, weak, slow pulse. The pale face and pale, flabby tongue result from the Deficient circulation of Qi and Xue to the tongue and to the face.

Deficient Shen Yang may or may not involve Deficient Jing. If it does, then there may also be signs of Deficient Jing, especially of the Yang aspect of Jing. Hence the sensation of cold is especially in the lumbar and knee regions, and there are problems of reproduction, and possibly of ears, teeth, etc. Shen is said to store the Will, and if Shen, and especially Shen Yang, is Deficient, this may lead to a lack of drive, either generally, hence the apathy, or in the specific case of reproduction, to a lack of sexual drive. The function of Yang is also to hold things in, and if Yang is Deficient, spermatorrhoea may occur, the leakage of sperm without erection or orgasm.

Deficient Shen Yang may result in failure to hold in urine, hence incontinence or frequency, or, especially if the Deficient Shen Yang is associated with Deficient Pi Yang, there may be failure to Transform and Transport Jin Ye properly, with consequential reduced urination and oedema. Deficient Pi Yang may also involve loss of appetite and loose stools. The general Deficiency of Qi and Xue, resulting from deficient Pi Yang, may result in malnutrition of the Muscles and hence in lassitude and general debility, weak pulse, and pale tongue with thin white coat.

Derivative Patterns
Deficiency of Shen Yang may involve one or more of four derivative patterns:-

Deficient Shen Jing (Yang)
Shen Qi not Firm
Shen Fails to Receive Qi
Water Overflowing

Deficient Shen Jing (Yang)
Each of the four derivative patterns has signs of Deficient Shen Yang, in addition to signs specific to itself. For example, Deficient Shen Jing (Yang) has the basic signs of Shen Yang Deficiency:- weakness and cold in lumbar region and knees; aversion to cold; deep, slow, weak pulse; and pale, flabby tongue with thin, white coat. In addition, Deficient Shen Jing (Yang), has signs concerned with reproduction and development, as discussed above.

Shen Qi not Firm
In addition to basic Deficient Shen Yang signs, this pattern has signs related to failure of the Yang function of holding in Jin Ye, as in incontinence of sperm or urine. There may be abundant, frequent urination, with incontinence, enuresis, and weak flow, or dribbling after urination. If the Deficient Shen Yang is associated with Deficient Pi Yang, there may be the inability of Yang to hold up the organs, with subsequent prolapse, see page 90.

Shen Fails to Receive Qi
In addition to basic Deficient Shen Yang signs, this pattern has signs related to the failure of Shen to hold down the Qi sent down by Fei in respiration. The Qi then rebels upwards resulting in difficult inhalation and shortness of breath aggravated by exertion, cough and asthma. Here, Deficient Shen Yang may also result in abundance or incontinence of urine, especially during asthma attack, due to inability of Shen Yang to hold the urine within Pang Guang. The close relationship of Shen and Fei in movement of Qi results in the tendency for Deficiency of Shen to result in Deficiency of Fei, and vice versa, so that often these two Patterns of Disharmony occur together.

Water Overflowing

In this pattern, there may be the simultaneous occurrence of four Yang Zang Deficiencies:-

Deficient Shen Yang
Deficient Pi Yang
Deficient Fei Yang
Deficient Xin Yang

In addition to the basic Shen Yang signs, there are those associated vwith insufficient Yang for proper Jin Ye metabolism and movement for example, reduced urination and oedema. If Shen Yang fails to support Pi Yang, then the failure of the Pi function of Transformation and Transportation of Jin Ye may result in distension of the abdomen by accumulation of fluids. If Shen Yang fails to support Fei Yang, then firstly there may be the signs of mutual weakness of Shen and Fei, described in the previous pattern, for example shortness of breath, cough and asthma. Secondly, there may be failure of the Shen and Fei functions of circulation of Jin Ye (see Figure 7.2 on page 69), resulting in copious watery sputum, oedema of the face, and general disruption of the harmony of Jin Ye. If Xin Yang Deficiency is also involved, there may be the combination of such signs as palpitation, shortness of breath and oedema.

This is a Deficiency pattern complicated by Excess, i.e. the Deficiency of Shen Yang is complicated by local Excess, specifically, the accumulation of Jin Ye.

Treatment

The principle of treatment is basically to strengthen and warm Shen Yang, using reinforcing method and moxa, and to treat whichever additional pattern predominates.

General Deficient Shen Yang

Taixi	KID.3	Strengthen Shen, and if moxa is used, strengthen Shen Yang.
Shenshu	BL.23	
Guanyuan	Ren 4	Strengthen Shen, especially Shen Yang.
Ming Men	Du 4	
Qihai	Ren 6	Strengthen circulation of Qi, especially if moxa is used; disperses Cold and Damp.

Deficient Jing Yang

In addition to the general points, points may be added depending on the predominant disharmony, for example Qixue, KID.13, and Zigong, (M-CA-18), for infertility.

Shen Qi not Firm

In enuresis, for example, Baihui, Du 20, and Sanyinjiao, SP6, can be added to the basic points. Baihui, especially with moxa, strengthens the Yang, and in particular, its ability to hold fluids in and organs up. Sanyinjiao, in this context, strengthens the Qi of the three Leg Yin Channels, thus helping Pang Guang to retain fluids.

Shen Fails to Receive Qi

In asthma, for example, points such as Shanzhong, Ren 17, Xuanji, Ren 21, and Tiantu, Ren 22, may be added to assist Rebellious Fei Qi to descend properly. Zusanli, ST.36, may be used to nourish Pi and Wei, and hence Shen.

Water Overflowing

In oedema, for example, such points as Sanyinjiao, SP.6, Yinlingquan, SP.9, and Shuifen, Ren 9, may be added to strengthen Qi and eliminate Damp. Weiyang, BL.53, the Lower He point of San Jiao, may be added to remove obstruction from the Water Passages. Pishu, BL.20, especially with moxa, can be added to warm and strengthen Pi Yang, to transform Jin Ye and eliminate Damp. Lieque, LU.7, and Feishu, BL.13, may be added to strengthen the Dispersing and Descending function of Fei; and Xinshu, BL.15, may be used with reinforcing method and moxa, to strengthen Xin Yang.

Common Disease Patterns

Patterns involving Deficient Shen Yang cover a very wide range indeed:- neurasthenia, adrenal or thyroid hypofunction, diabetes insipidus, lumbago, chronic nephritis, incontinence, impotence, infertility, asthma, emphysema, pulmonary heart disease, cardiac insufficiency, oedema and chronic diarrhoea, chronic ear disorders.

Deficient Shen Yin

Signs

General	malar flush, thirst, constipation, dark urine,
Deficient Yin	palms and soles hot, night sweats
Deficient Jing (Yin)	sore knees and back, tenderness, dizziness, poor memory, nocturnal emissions with dreams, premature ejaculation
Pulse	thin and rapid
Tongue	red with no coat, perhaps with cracks

Pathology

Symptoms here are those of Deficient Yin and of Heat, and of Deficient Shen Jing, especially of its Yin aspects. Which of these categories of signs predominates, will depend on the situation. For example, if Jin Ye are severely damaged by Heat and Dryness, the Deficient Shen Yin may progress to Blazing Shen Fire condition, sometimes listed as a separate Pattern of Disharmony, with signs of more severe Heat, especially in the upper Body. The Heat and Dryness associated with Yin Deficiency results in such signs as thin body, thirst, thin rapid pulse, and thin red tongue with little coat.

If the Yang aspect of Jing is the predominant Deficiency, then, as stated above, there may be reduced sexual desire, impotence and leakage of sperm without erection or orgasm. If the Yin aspect of Jing is the predominant deficiency, then there may be mental, physical and sexual restlessness and over-excitability. This may result in premature ejaculation, and in noctural emission with dream-disturbed or restless sleep. However, though this may seem an Excess condition, compared to the pattern of the Deficient Yang aspect of Jing, which is more obviously a Deficiency, nevertheless both conditions are based on Deficiency. Therefore, although the Yin Deficiency may give rise to sexual hyperactivity, this will only further aggravate the underlying Deficiency of Yin and of Jing.

Sweating

The sweating resulting from Deficient Yin must be differentiated from the sweating resulting from Deficient Yang. In chronic Deficiency conditions, sweating may occur in the daytime with or without exercise, or in the night. Daytime sweating may mean Wei Qi is not properly regulating the pores, and holding Jin Ye inside the Body, due to Deficiency of Qi, especially Deficiency of Yang. Yang Deficiency will be most apparent in the daytime, the time of greatest activity of Yang, hence daytime sweating. At night, when Yin should be dominant, and the Body less active, if there is not enough Yin to control the Heat, the latter may cause the pores to open, resulting in night-time sweating. Sweating due to Deficient Yin will tend to be accompanied by signs of Heat, and sweating due to Deficient Yang will tend to be accompanied by signs of Cold.

Treatment

The principle of treatment is to strengthen Yin, using reinforcing method but no moxa, and to pacify Fire, if this is Blazing, using reducing method, and to attend to any other patterns that may predominate. Such points as the following may be used:-

Taixi	KID.3	Strengthens Shen, and in this case, Shen Yin.
Shenshu	BL.23	Strengthens Shen, and in this case may disperse heat in the Lower Jiao.
Guanyuan	Ren 4	Strengthens Shen, and though especially used for Deficiency of Shen Yang, can also strengthen Shen Yin in this case.
Zhoahai	KID.6	Strengthens Shen Yin, eliminates Heat.
Sanyinjiao	SP.6	Strengthens Yin of Shen and Gan; together with Lieque, LU.7, strengthens Yin of Shen and Fei.
Yongquan	KID.1 ⎫	May be added to pacify Fire, and Yongquan
Rangu	KID.2 ⎭	especially to calm Shen* and Hyperactive Yang of Gan and Xin.

In addition to these general points, points may be added depending on the particular disharmony manifested by a particular patient. For example, in essential hypertension of the Deficient Yin - Hyperactive Yang type, the following points may be added:-

Fengchi	GB.20	Pacifies Hyperactive Yang.
Quchi	LI.11 ⎱	Both on Yang channels, may be used to drain
Zusanli	ST.36 ⎰	Excess from Yang channels.
Taichong	LIV.3	Pacifies Hyperactive Gan Yang and Wind.

Common Disease Patterns

As with Deficient Shen Yang, the patterns of Deficient Shen Yin cover a wide range of disease categories:- essential hypertension, tachycardia, hyper- thyroidism, diabetis mellitus, lumbago, chronic nephritis, chronic urogenital infections, menstrual problems, pulmonary T.B., and chronic ear problems.

Summary

The Shen function of storing Jing is of fundamental importance to the Body. Deficient Shen Jing results in disharmonies of birth, growth, development, reproduction, Bones, Brain, ears and hair.

Since Shen is the foundation of Yin Yang within the Body, relative Deficiency of Shen Yin or Shen Yang may affect the balance Yin Yang in the other Zang Fu. Hence patterns of Deficient Shen Yin or Deficient Shen Yang are often found in association with one or more patterns of Deficiency of Yin or Yang of other Zang Fu.

There is a close association between the Shen function of Ruling the Water, and the activities of the other Zang Fu involved in Jin Ye metabolism. Hence, Shen Deficiency is likely to be associated with disharmony of these other Zang Fu in this context.

There is a close association in respiration between Fei that sends down the Qi, and Shen that holds it down. Deficient Shen Qi and Deficient Fei Qi are often associated.

The very close association between Shen and Pang Guang leads to the common association of this Zang Fu pair in Patterns of Disharmony, and to the use of points on Shen Jing Luo to treat disharmonies of Pang Guang, and conversely, the use of points on Pang Guang Jing Luo to treat disharmonies of Shen.

Table 7.1 Shen Patterns of Disharmony

Pattern	Symptoms	Pulse	Tongue
Deficient Shen Jing	lumbar soreness; weak knees; retarded growth; infertility; loose teeth; greying hair; poor memory; dizziness; tinnitus	deep weak	various
Deficient Shen Yang	lumbar soreness; weak knees; sensations of cold; impotence & reduced sexual drive	deep slow weak	pale, flabby; thin white coat
Shen Qi not Firm	as for Deficient Shen Yang; plus enuresis & spermat-orrhoea	deep slow weak	pale, flabby; thin white coat
Shen Fails to Receive Qi	as for Deficient Shen Yang; plus asthma, shortness of breath, cough	deep slow weak	pale, flabby; thin white coat
Water Overflowing	as for Shen Fails to Receive Qi; ± reduced urination, oedema; copious, thin sputum; palpitations	deep	pale
Deficient Shen Yin	lumbar soreness; weak knees; malar flush; thirst; premature ejaculation	thin rapid	red ± cracks; no coat
Damp Heat in Pang Guang	difficult, painful urination with retention or frequency; thirst; ± fever; lumbar soreness	rapid slippery	red; yellow greasy coat

Pang Guang

Functions

There is a very close relationship between Shen and its paired Fu, Pang Guang. The latter receives, stores and transforms fluids prior to their excretion from the Body as urine. The Fluid received by Pang Guang is the impure fraction received by Shen from Fei, and from Xiao Chang and Da Chang. The ability of Pang Guang to retain and transform the fluids depends on Shen Qi and especially on Shen Yang. If these are Deficient, Pang Guang cannot properly retain the Fluids and there may be enuresis, incontinence, etc., alternatively, there may be difficulty in urination with retention of urine.

Since the primary function of San Jiao is Jin Ye movement and metabolism, there is a functional link between Pang Guang and the Lower Jiao especially. If there is failure of the function of San Jiao to allow free movement of Jin Ye, i.e. if the Water Passages become obstructed, Damp may accumulate, and on stagnation, may become Damp Heat. This may be aggravated if there is also Depression of Gan Qi, and if there is Heat, especially Damp Heat, in Gan and Dan channels. Also, if Xin Fire moves downwards into Xiao Chang, this Heat can move into Pang Guang, giving a pathological link between Pang Guang, Xiao Chang and Xin.

Hence, via the metabolism and movement of Jin Ye, Pang Guang is linked in physiology and pathology with all the other Zang Fu.

Patterns of Disharmony

The most important pattern is that of Damp Heat in Pang Guang, which is sometimes divided into various sub-categories. Some texts also list the category of Deficient Pang Guang Qi, but this has already been dealt with in this book under the heading of Deficient Shen Yang.

Damp Heat in Pang Guang

Signs
Signs will vary depending on whether the pattern is based on Deficiency or Excess, on which Zang Fu disharmonies predominate, and on the preponderance of Heat or Cold, Deficient Yin or Deficient Yang in the particular patient. For example, if the Damp condenses to Phlegm, the action of Heat on the Phlegm may give rise to stones.

Generally, there may be cloudy urine, perhaps with blood or stones. Urination may be frequent, difficult, urgent or painful. There may be signs of Heat such as thirst, fever, rapid pulse and red tongue with yellow coat; and there may be signs of Damp, such as slippery pulse and greasy tongue coat.

Origins
As shown in Figure 7.4, Depression of Gan Qi, Deficient San Jiao, Deficient Fei Qi, Deficient Pi Yang, or invasion of External Cold and Damp, may originate

stagnation of Damp. Deficient Shen Qi may interact with deficient Fe Qi as described above. Deficient Shen Yang may contribute to Deficient Pi Yang, and may facilitate the invasion of External Cold and Damp. Chronic retention of Cold and Damp in the Lower Jiao can eventually injure Shen Yang, just as long-term retention of Damp Heat can injure Shen Yin.

Figure 7.4 Origins of Damp Heat in Pang Guang

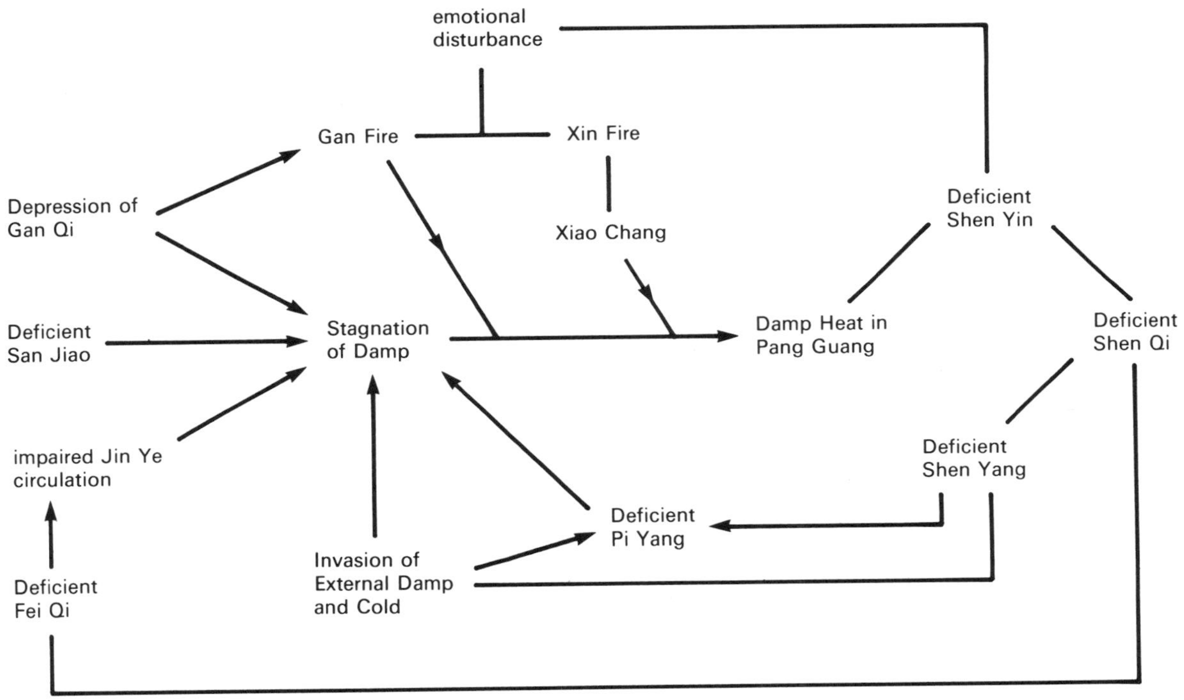

Depression of Gan Qi may give rise to Gan Fire, and emotional disturbance may originate or aggravate Gan and Xin Fire, and also Deficient Shen, Gan, and Xin Yin. The resultant Heat may then move downwards to affect Pang Guang, originating or aggravating the condition of Damp Heat.

Treatment
The principle of treatment is to spread Pang Guang Qi, clearing Damp Heat from the Lower Jiao; and to treat any additional disharmonies. The method of treatment may be reducing method, even method, or reinforcing method, depending on the situation, and on the points used:-

Shenshu	BL.23	Strengthens Shen and regulates the passage of water, especially in the Lower Jiao.
Pangguangshu	BL.28	Strengthens Pang Guang and disperses the Qi of the Lower Jaio.

Zhongji	Ren 3	Alarm point of Pang Guang, and intersection of three leg Yin Channels with Ren channel. Disperses Damp Heat in Lower Jiao.
Sanyinjiao	SP.6	Regulates Shen and Gan and strengthens Pi.
Yinlingquan	SP.9	Disperses stagnation in the Lower Jiao, especially of Damp Heat.

All these points clear Damp and Heat from Pang Guang and the Lower Jiao. In the case of a predominantly Excess condition, these points would be used with reducing or even method.

Common Disease Patterns
In this pattern of Damp Heat in Pang Guang, are included cystitis, prostatitis, bladder stones, and general inflammatory diseases of the bladder and urinary tract.

Chapter
8

Pi (Spleen) and Wei (Stomach)

Pi

Functions

1. Rules Tansformation and Transportation
2. Rules the Muscles and the Limbs
3. Governs Xue
4. Holds up the Organs
5. Opens into the Mouth; Manifests in the Lips

After Shen, the foundation of the prenatal energies of the Body, Pi is considered, since it is the foundation of postnatal life.

Rules Transformation and Transportation

Under the influence of Pi, the digestion products of food and drink are separated into relatively pure and impure fractions. The latter passes via Xiao Chang to Da Chang and Pang Guang for final absorption and excretion. The pure fraction is sent up by Pi to Fei, where it is converted into Qi, Xue, and Jin Ye; see Figure 3.6, page 18.

If Pi function is harmonious, there are sufficient Qi, Xue and Jin Ye for the needs of the Body. If Transformation and Transportation is impaired, i.e. Pi function is Deficient, then there may be Deficient Qi and Deficient Xue, and possible accumulation and stagnation of Jin Ye as Damp and Phlegm. Also, since Pi is the main digestive organ in TCM, there may be a variety of alimentary disharmonies.

Rules the Muscles and the Limbs

If the Pi function of digestion and movement, Transportation and Transformation, is harmonious there is a good supply of Qi and Xue, and these Substances are adequately transported to the Muscles, so that the Muscles are full and firm and the limbs warm and energised for movement. If there is Deficient and inadequate Transportation of Qi and Xue, the Muscles are not properly nourished, lose their tone, and become thin, wasted or even atrophied. The limbs become weak and cold, and the Body lethargic.

There is considerable overlap between the concept of Muscles ruled by Pi, and the concept of Tendons, ruled by Gan. This is discussed on page 173.

Governs Xue

In addition to its vital role in the formation of Xue, Pi governs Xue in the sense of holding it within its proper pathways. If Pi Qi, and especially Pi Yang, is Deficient, and Xue is not held in Xue Mai, it leaks out as haemorrhages of various kinds, for example melaena, petechiae, menorrhagia.

Holds up the Organs

Another restraining function of Pi Yang is that of helping to hold the organs up and within the Body. If there is Deficiency of Pi Yang, there may be prolapse of various organs, especially in the lower Body, for example uterus, anus, bladder, stomach and kidneys.

Opens into the Mouth; Manifests in the Lips

If Pi Qi is abundant, the mouth can differentiate the Five Flavours and the lips are red and moist. If Pi Qi is Deficient, there may be loss of taste, and the lips may be pale and dry. If there is Heat in Pi and Wei, the lips may be dry and cracked.

Fluids, Damp and Phlegm

Pi governs the proper Transformation and Transportation of Jin Ye and is part of the cycle of Jin Ye metabolism, see Figure 7.2 page 69. If Pi is Deficient, Jin Ye may not be transformed properly and may become impure or turbid. Also, if the Transportation of Jin Ye is defective, they may accumulate, forming oedema and Damp. If Damp stagnates it may form Damp Heat, and if turbid Jin Ye stagnates, it may condense and become Phlegm.

The idea of Phlegm or Mucus, Tan in TCM, is different from the Western concept. Damp is wet, slow, heavy and lingering, but Phlegm is heavier and thicker than Damp, and even more likely to cause obstruction and blockage. Phlegm is both the result and the cause of disharmony.

Phlegm is a progression of Damp, and is usually associated with it. Phlegm is generally related to Pi Deficiency, and especially with the association of Deficient Pi Yang and Deficient Shen Yang. Pi is said to form Phlegm, and Fei to store it. Phlegm may be both cause and result of the failure of the Dispersing function of Fei, giving rise to catarrh in chest, throat, nose and sinuses; see page 146. Phlegm in the throat can give rise to the sensation of 'lump in the throat', the 'Plumseed Qi' sensation of TCM; this is associated with Depression of Gan Qi, see page 106.

Depression of Gan Qi may also be involved in the stagnation that results in the condensation of Phlegm as sub- cutaneous lumps, lymphadenopathy or goitre. These condensations of Phlegm then cause further obstruction and blockage.

Phlegm Damp refers to the presence of Phlegm and Damp; Phlegm Cold refers to the presence of Phlegm combined with Internal or External Cold; and Phlegm Heat or Phlegm Fire refers to the combination of Phlegm and Internal or External Heat. If Phlegm stagnates for long periods it may give rise to Phlegm Heat, just as Damp may become Damp Heat. Phlegm Wind is the combination of the factors of Phlegm and Internal Wind.

Figure 8.1 Types of Phlegm

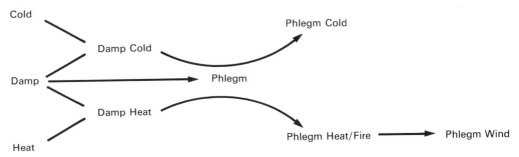

Phlegm may combine with External Wind and Cold, as in facial paralysis, to obstruct the flow of Qi and Xue, resulting in malnutrition of Jing Luo. In Windstroke, Phlegm may combine with Internal Gan Wind and Heat to disrupt Jing Luo causing hemiplegia. If Phlegm obstructs the Orifices of Xin, then Shen* is Disturbed, and there may be signs of mania, depression or loss of consciousness, see page 133. If Phlegm rebels upwards, the Qi in the head may become disorderly, with obstruction of the Orifices of the Senses, and the patient may become dizzy or lose consciousness, as in epilepsy. In obstruction of the Orifices of Xin or of the Senses, Phlegm is often combined with Fire and Internal Wind, from Blazing Xin Fire, Blazing Gan Fire, or from general fever; see page 116.

Both Damp and Phlegm are usually accompanied by the signs of slippery pulse and greasy tongue coat; the differentiation between Damp and Phlegm usually depends on the other associated signs.

Patterns of Disharmony

Deficient Pi Qi
Deficient Pi Yang
Inability of Pi to Govern Xue
Sinking of Pi Qi
Invasion of Pi by Cold and Damp
Damp Heat Accumulates in Pi
Turbid Phlegm Disturbing the Head

The foundations of Pi disharmony are the tendency of Pi to Deficiency of Qi and Yang, and its proneness to invasion by Damp and Cold.

Pi disharmonies are generally of Deficiency. However, Deficiency of Pi Qi and Yang may result in poor Transformation and Transportation of Jin Ye and hence an accumulation of Damp, forming oedema, whether local or general. This may be termed Deficiency turning into Excess, or, more accurately, Excess with underlying Deficiency. Only when there is invasion of Pi by External Damp Cold or Damp Heat, is there anything approaching a true Excess condition, and even then, the invasion may be predisposed by underlying Deficiency of Pi Qi and Pi Yang.

Origins

Deficiency of Prenatal Qi can result in Deficiency of Postnatal Qi; Shen Qi Deficiency can give rise to Pi Qi Deficiency; and congenital weakness of Shen and Pi can originate Pi Qi Deficiency. Any chronic disease that weakens either the Body in general, or the digestion in particular, will originate Deficiency of Pi Qi. Traditionally, excessive work, worry or study weaken Pi Qi; as does Invasion of Pi by Gan Qi, see page 106.

Inadequate nutrition, over-eating, eating at irregular times, or the consumption of food to which the system is unaccustomed, can give rise to Deficient Pi Qi over a period of time. Excess spicy, greasy food and alcohol can contribute to a variety of disharmonies, including Damp Heat in Pi, Damp Heat in Gan, and Blazing Wei Fire. Excessive intake of raw or cold food and drink can aggravate Deficient Pi Yang, or result in Invasion of Pi by External Cold and Damp. Obviously, in nutrition, what is inadequate or excessive for one person may not be for another. Nutritional requirements depend on the individual, at a particular age, and in a given set of circumstances. Nevertheless, gross inadequacy, excess, or irregularity are bound to damage Pi Qi eventually.

External Cold and Damp, or less commonly, External Heat and Damp, may invade Pi. Invasion of Pi by Cold and Damp may be facilitated by, or give rise to Deficient Pi Yang. Deficient Pi Qi and Yang may precipitate Failure of Pi to Govern Xue, Sinking of Pi Qi, or Deficiency of the Pi function of Transformation and Transportation. The last mentioned pattern may cause Deficiency of Qi and Xue, and accumulation and turbidity of Jin Ye, leading to accumulation of Damp, which may condense as Phlegm.

Deficiency of Pi Qi

Signs

Loss of appetite, anorexia, slight abdominal pain and distension that are relieved on pressure, oedema, loose stools, thin muscles, weak limbs, general lassitude, sallow complexion, empty pulse, and pale flabby tongue with thin white coat.

Pathology

The signs of Deficient Pi Qi are basically signs of Deficient Qi, Deficient Xue, Jin Ye disharmony, and weakness of the digestive system. This is essentially a Deficiency pattern, even when poor Transformation and Transportation of Jin Ye lead to a local accumulation and Excess of Damp. Weakness of Pi results in poor digestion, loss of appetite and anorexia. Diarrhoea and loose stools, especially loose stools containing particles of undigested food, derive from weakness of digestive

Figure 8.2   Origins of Pi Disharmonies

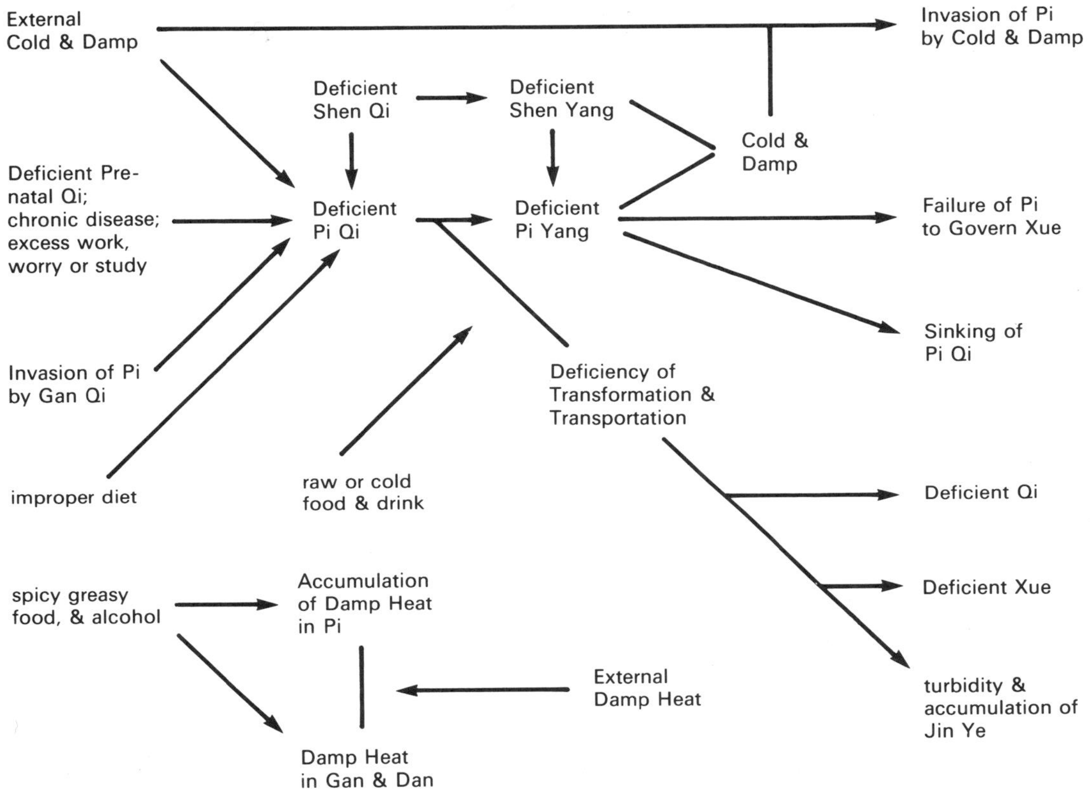

function of Pi, from poor Transformation and Transportation of Jin Ye and from failure of Pi Qi and Pi Yang to hold things in and up. Abdominal distension and oedema result from failure of Pi function of Transformation and Transportation of Jin Ye. Abdominal pain that is relieved on pressure, reflects a Deficiency condition. Thin Muscles, weak limbs, lassitude, pale or sallow face, empty pulse, and pale flabby tongue reflect the Deficiencies of Qi and Xue, which are insufficient to fill and nourish the Muscles, Flesh and Jing Luo.

The tongue coat is a manifestation of the activity of Pi. In the Transformation of food into pure essences, small amounts of impurities rise upwards and collect on the tongue. A thin coat represents either normality or Deficiency. A white coat reflects either External or Internal Cold. In this case, the thin white coat reflects the Deficiency of Pi function.

Treatment

The principle of treatment is to strengthen Pi Qi, using reinforcing method and often moxa also. For example, in a case of generalised digestive weakness, with the signs described above, points such as the following could be used:-

Zusanli	ST.36	To strengthen function of Pi and Wei, to strengthen formation and circulation of Qi and Xue, and hence to strengthen both digestive and general weakness.
Zhongwan	Ren 12	To strengthen and regulate Qi of Pi and Wei, to eliminate Damp.
Pishu	BL.20	To promote Transformation and Transformation and function of Pi, and eliminate Damp.

These are the three basic points, but of course the choice of points would be varied according to the particular requirement of the patient.

Common disease patterns
General weakness, anaemia, general digestive weakness, chronic gastritis, gastric or duodenal ulcer, chronic diarrhoea. This pattern may also be involved in some forms of myasthenia.

Deficient Pi Yang

Signs
Signs of this pattern are as for Deficient Pi Qi, but also include signs of Cold, for example cold limbs, aversion to cold, abdominal pain relieved by heat as well as pressure, undigested food in watery stools, greater tendency to retention of urine and oedema. The pulse may be deep and slow as well as weak, and the tongue may have a white coat that is thicker than in the case of Deficient Pi Qi, and which may even be greasy.

Pathology
In addition to signs of Deficiency and weakness of Pi, in this pattern there are also signs of Cold, due to Deficient Yang. Deficient Pi Yang is often a progression of Deficient Pi Qi, and the signs may be more severe. For example, the undigested food in watery stools reflects a greater degree of weakness of Transformation and Transportation of both food and Jin Ye. Similarly, the thicker white or greasy white tongue coat reflects both the Internal Cold and the greater Deficiency of Transformation and Transportation of Jin Ye, with accumulation of Damp and perhaps Phlegm. The additional pulse qualities of depth and slowness reflect the insufficiency of Yang to raise and move the Qi of the Body and the pulse.

Treatment
The principle of treatment is to strengthen and warm Pi Yang by reinforcing method and moxa. Points used are as for Deficient Pi Qi, but the emphasis on moxa. If Deficient Pi Yang is associated with Deficient Shen Yang , points such as Shenshu, BL.23, Mingmen, Du 4, and Guanyuan, Ren 4, may also be used with reinforcing method and moxa, to strengthen Shen Yang, and hence the Yang of the entire Body, and of Pi in particular.

Common Disease Patterns
These are as for Deficient Pi Qi, but in this case, the signs would tend to be more severe, and include signs of Cold, and possibly of Deficient Shen Yang, for

example oedema and urinary retention. However, separation of Deficient Pi Qi and Deficient Pi Yang is rather arbitrary, since they are so closely related, often occurring together in practice.

Inability of Pi to Govern Xue

Signs
These may include some signs of Deficient Pi Qi or Deficient Pi Yang, and in addition haemorrhages, especially of the lower Body, for example, purpura, melaena and abnormal uterine bleeding.

Pathology
These signs result from Deficiency of Qi and Deficiency of Yang of Pi, resulting in insufficient Qi and Yang to hold Xue in Xue Mai, with resultant extravasation. This type of haemorrhage is associated with Deficiency and with signs of Cold, contrasting with the type of haemorrhage associated with Excess and with Heat, as in Gan disharmonies.

Treatment
The principle of treatment is to strengthen Pi Qi and to strengthen and warm Pi Yang, to enable Pi Qi and Pi Yang to govern Xue. Also, Shen Yang is strengthened and warmed to support Pi Yang. Reinforcing method and moxa are used; for example in abnormal uterine bleeding, four important points are:-
Guanyuan, Ren 4, Sanyinjiao, SP.6, Shenshu, BL.23, Jiaoxin, KID.8.

These four points strengthen Pi and Shen, and regulate Chong Mai and Ren Mai, to govern Xue. The combination of Guanyuan and Sanyinjiao can invigorate Shen, Pi, Gan, Ren Mai and Chong Mai to restore the function of the storage and control of Xue. Shenshu and Jiaoxin, invigorate the Shen Yang function of astringency, of holding Xue within Xue Mai. Jiaoxin is an empirical point in this context. Contrast these points with the points used for abnormal uterine bleeding with signs of Heat and Excess, see page 109.

The following points may be added as required, and used with reinforcing method and moxa:-

Quihai	Ren 6	To invigorate Qi and Yang.
Zusanli	ST.36 }	To reduce bleeding by strengthening Pi function
Pishu	BL.20 }	
Geshu	BL.17	The Influential point for Xue.
Ming Men	Du 4 }	To strengthen Yang Qi.
Fuliu	KID.7 }	

Further points may be added depending on the accompanying signs, and the needs of the particular patient at that time.

Common Disease Patterns
Functional abnormal uterine bleeding, bleeding haemorrhoids, haemophilia.

Sinking of Pi Qi

Signs
The pattern of Sinking of Pi Qi may show some signs of Deficient Pi Qi and of Deficient Pi Yang, and, in addition prolapse of internal organs of the lower Body. For example, prolapse of anus, vagina, uterus, bladder and stomach, with dragging sensation in the lower abdomen. Also there may be signs of severe chronic diarrhoea or urinary incontinence.

Pathology
The signs result from the failure of the function of Yang and Qi to hold things up.

Treatment
The principle of treatment is to strengthen Qi and Yang, especially of Shen and Pi, and to use points specific for prolapse of the particular organ or organs involved. For example, there are various methods for treating stomach prolapse; most involving transverse insertion of long needles into the abdominal muscle layer,often joining two or more points together. Points such as the following may be used:- Weishangxue, N-C-A-18, Guanyuan, Ren 4, Quihai, Ren 6, Zhongwan, Ren 12, and Zusanli, ST.36. Zusanli and Zhongwan are used with reinforcing method and moxa, to strengthen the Middle Jiao.

Common Disease Patterns
This pattern includes prolapse of the organs of the lower Body, haemorrhage, diarrhoea and urinary incontinence.

Invasion of Pi by Cold and Damp

Origins
External Cold may enter the Body either as the Climatic Factor, or via excess intake of raw or cold food and drink. Such things as iced water, ice- cream, and food and drink straight from the refrigerator, are likely to depress the function of Pi, whether they are taken in winter or in summer, and according to TCM, should be avoided.

External Damp may become a pathological factor, especially in a rural society, as mist or fog. This may occur in mountainous areas, over stretches of water, or in the early morning before sunrise, and may be a hazard for those working in these conditions. Damp may also be a factor for those working in water, for those working or living in a damp place, or for those who, after profuse perspiration, remain in damp clothes.

Invasion of Cold and Damp, unless the Body is chronically exposed to extreme levels of these factors, only occurs when the Body is weak, either due to constitution, or to the effects of other disease factors, for example trauma, overwork and emotional disturbance.

Either Cold or Damp may eventually give rise to Deficient Yang, which itself may give rise to Internal Cold, due to lack of the Yang capacity to warm and move; or to Internal Damp, due to inadequate Transformation and Transportation of function of Pi, leading to accumulation of Jin Ye. Cold and Damp may therefore give rise to each other, via Deficient Yang. Thus Internal Cold and Internal Damp often occur together in the Body, just as External Cold and External Damp are a common combination of External Disease Factors.

Sub-divisions

The pattern of Invasion of Pi by Cold and Damp may be sub-divided according to whether Cold or Damp predominates. If the former, a common association is with the pattern of Retention of Fluid in Wei due to Cold, see page 97, and with the pattern of Deficient Pi Yang, see page 88.

If Damp predominates, sub-division is according to whether the Damp is predominantly Internal or External. The Internal pattern is sometimes called **Damp Distressing Pi**, and the External pattern is sometimes called **External Damp Obstructing**. The origin of these two patterns is summarized in Figure 8.3.

Deficient Shen Yang may underlie or accompany Deficient Pi Yang, and both may give rise to Internal Cold and Damp. Alternatively, Internal Cold and Damp may, over a long period, give rise to Deficient Shen Yang and Deficient Pi Yang. This Internal Cold and Damp may invade Pi. This is a Deficiency pattern turning into Excess, and is usually a chronic disharmony with a gradual onset.

External Cold and Damp may invade Pi, an External pattern which is usually acute and of more sudden onset than the pattern of Deficiency. However, Deficient Pi Yang and Deficient Shen Yang may predispose towards Invasion of Pi by External Cold and Damp, so that both the Internal and External patterns may occur together. For example, there may be an acute aggravation of the chronic Deficiency condition by the Invasion of External Cold and Damp, resulting in a temporary Excess situation.

Figure 8.3 Origin of Damp Disharmonies of Pi

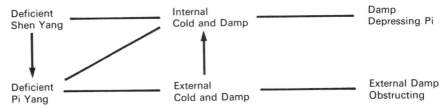

Signs

These may include lethargy, loss of appetite and sense of taste, feelings of heaviness of limbs or head, and feelings of fullness in chest or abdomen. There may be copious or turbid secretions, for example, cloudy urine, leucorrhoea, diarrhoea, stickiness of eyes and fluid-filled skin eruptions. There may be retention or dribbling of urine and oedema. The pulse is slippery and perhaps slow; the tongue is pale with thick white greasy coat.

Pathology

The signs of this pattern may include signs of Deficient Pi Qi and Deficient Pi Yang, but are characterised by signs of Damp. Some signs of Damp derive from the accumulation and turbidity of Jin Ye resulting from poor Transformation and Transportation function of Pi. Also, Damp is associated with accumulation, and may result in obstruction and stagnation. For example, obstruction of the movement of Qi results in the feelings of fullness in chest and abdomen, and incomplete urination. The turbidity of Jin Ye leads to cloudy urine, stickiness of the eyes, etc; and the simple accumulation of fluid results in oedema, fluid-filled skin eruptions and in diarrhoea.

The slippery pulse is associated with Damp or Phlegm in the system, and the slow pulse with Cold. The pale tongue is associated with Deficient Pi Qi and Pi Yang, the thick greasy coat with Internal Damp or Phlegm, and the white coat with Cold.

Some signs are due to Damp depressing the function of Spleen, for example in general lethargy, loss of appetite and loss of ability of Pi to distinguish the Five Flavours.

Treatment
The principle of treatment is to strengthen Pi and Wei to resolve Damp, and to warm and strengthen Qi and Yang to disperse Cold. All the points are used with both reinforcing method and moxa. For example, for chronic enteritis caused by Invasion of Pi by Cold and Damp, the following points may be used:-

Qihai	Ren 6	Strengthens Qi so as to retain fluids, but also invigorates Qi circulation to disperse Damp.
Zhongwan	Ren 12	Invigorates Pi Qi and Pi Yang, to aid Transformation and Transportation functions of Pi.
Tianshu	ST.25	Regulates Qi of Wei and intestines; when used together with Zhongwan, invigorates Pi and reduces Damp.
Shangjuxu	ST.37	Lower He point of Da Chang, regulates Qi of Wei and intestines, invigorates Pi and reduces Damp.

Common Disease Patterns
This pattern includes chronic gastro-enteritis, dysentery or hepatitis.

Damp Heat Accumulates in Pi

This pattern may be sub-divided according to whether Damp or Heat predominate. If the former, there will be no thirst, or thirst without desire to drink; a pulse that is not particularly rapid, and a tongue that is not particularly red. In the latter, there will be thirst, the pulse will be rapid, and tongue will be red.

The pattern may also be sub-divided according to whether the Damp Heat is predominantly External or predominantly Internal. The latter is generally chronic and of gradual onset, and can arise from excess consumption of greasy foods, alcohol, etc., over a long period of time. The former is generally acute and of sudden onset, and can arise from either exposure to hot humid climate, or from consumption of contaminated food.

A further sub-division can be made according to whether obstruction of the flow of bile occurs or not. If it does not, then the signs and treatment of this pattern are similar to those of Blazing Wei Fire, see page 99. If there is obstruction of bile, resulting in jaundice and bitter taste in the mouth, then the signs and treatment are similar to those of Damp Heat in Gan and Dan, see page 118.

Signs of Heat are not usually associated with Pi, and some texts do not include the category of Damp Heat Accumulating in Pi; the Common Disease Patterns of hepatitis, cholecystitis and cirrhosis generally being included under Damp Heat in Gan and Dan.

Signs

There may be loss of appetite, general lethargy, sensation of heaviness or distension, low fever, thirst with no desire to drink; scanty, slightly yellow urine; jaundice, and bitter taste in the mouth. The tongue may be slightly red with a thick greasy yellowish coat; and the pulse may be slippery and slightly rapid.

Pathology

There are signs of Damp accumulating and obstructing flow of Qi, such as sensations of heaviness or distension, and scanty urination. There are signs of Damp depressing the Pi function, for example loss of appetite and general lethargy. There are signs of Heat, for example low fever, moderate thirst, slightly yellow urine, slightly rapid pulse and slightly red tongue with yellowish coat. Jaundice and bitter taste in the mouth may be present if the flow of bile is obstructed. Slippery pulse and thick, greasy tongue coat represent an accumulation of Damp within the Body.

Treatment

See page 118, for treatment of hepatitis due to accumulation of Damp Heat in Gan and Dan, and see page 99, for treatment of stomach ulcer due to Blazing Wei Fire.

Common Disease Patterns

This pattern includes acute or chronic gastro-enteritis, acute hepatitis, cholecystitis and cirrhosis.

Turbid Phlegm Disturbing the Head

This pattern is a particular development of Pi Damp. Since Phlegm is heavier than Damp, the pattern is characterised by severe dizziness, rather than by sensations of heaviness in the head. It is associated with the category of hypertension corresponding to obstruction by Phlegm and Damp; involving limbs heavy and numb with clumsy movement, congested feeling of chest, palpitation, dizziness, nausea and vomiting, slippery pulse, and tongue with thick greasy coat.

In addition to general points for hypertension such as Fengchi, GB.20, Quchi,

LI.11, Zusanli, ST.36, and Taichong, LIV.3; the following points are added to dispel Excess Phlegm and Damp:- Neiguan, P.6, Fenglong, ST.40, and Yinglingquan, SP.9.

Fengchi	GB.20 ⎱	Pacify Gan Yang and Gan Wind and calm
Taichong	LIV.3 ⎰	the mind.
Quchi	CO.11 ⎱	In this context, eliminates Wind and
Zusanli	ST.36 ⎰	regulates the circulation of Qi and Xue and drains Excess from Yang channels.
Fenglong	ST.40	Transforms Phlegm.
Neiguan	P.6	Opens chest, calms Xin and mind, and pacifies Wei.
Yinglinquan	SP.9	Eliminates Damp and obstructions.

This pattern is not included by some texts, and is not given separate importance in this book. Disharmonies involving obstruction of the Orifices of Xin, or the Orifices or the Senses by Phlegm, are included in such disease patterns as Windstroke sequellae (see page 114), mania (see page 132), and epilepsy (see page 114).

Summary

The Patterns of Disharmony of Pi are basically patterns of Deficiency, specifically of Deficient Qi and of Deficient Yang. Particular progressions of Deficient Pi Qi

Table 8.1 Pi Patterns of Disharmony

Pattern	Signs	Pulse	Tongue
Deficient Pi Qi	general lassitude; muscular weakness; sallow complexion loss of appetite; anorexia; abdominal distension; oedema; loose stools	empty	pale, flabby; thin white coat
Deficient Pi Yang	as for Deficient Pi Qi; plus cold & pain in abdomen, alleviated by warmth; chilly limbs	empty slow deep	as above, white coat
Inability of Pi to Govern Xue	as for Deficient Pi Qi; plus purpura; rectal or uterine bleeding	empty	as above
Sinking of Pi Qi	as for Deficient Pi Qi; plus prolapse of anus, uterus or stomach; chronic diarrhoea	empty	as above
Invasion of Pi by Cold & Damp	as for Deficient Pi Qi, plus heaviness of limbs & head; fullness of chest & abdomen; retention of urine; leukorrhoea	slippery slow	pale; thick white greasy coat
Damp Heat Accumulates in Pi	feeling of fullness in chest and/or abdomen; thirst without desire to drink; scanty yellowish urine; ± jaundice & bitter taste	slippery slightly rapid	reddish; thick yellowish coat

94

and Deficient Pi Yang are the Sinking of Pi Qi and the Inability of Pi to Govern Xue. Deficient Pi Qi and Deficient Pi Yang may be aggravated by or may be predisposed to Invasion of Pi by External Cold and Damp. Differentiation between signs of Damp and signs of Cold is, for example, between sensations of heaviness or sensations of pain, aversion to Damp or aversion to Cold, a pulse which is predominantly slippery or a pulse which is predominantly slow, and a tongue which is greasy or is not. Invasion of Pi by External Cold and Damp may give rise to an Excess pattern, or if there is an underlying Deficiency of Pi Qi and of Pi Yang, to a situation of Deficiency turning into Excess. Some texts list another Excess pattern, that of Accumulation of Damp Heat in Pi. Other texts do not list this category which may be included in Damp Heat in Gan and Dan. The pattern of Turbid Phlegm Disturbing the Head, is also a pattern which is listed in some texts but not in others.

Various Pi disharmonies may occur together, for example Deficient Pi Qi, Deficient Pi Yang and Invasion of Pi by Cold and Damp. Also, Pi disharmonies may be associated with disharmonies of other Zang Fu, for example Deficient Shen Yang may be associated with Deficient Pi Yang, Invasion of Pi by Gan may be associated with Deficient Pi Qi, and Invasion of Pi by Cold and Damp may be associated with Retention of Fluid in Wei due to Cold. For a further discussion on these relationships, see pages 203-204.

Wei

Wei is the Fu system that is traditionally linked with Pi. The association with Pi and Wei is very close, and there is considerable overlap in both physiology and pathology.

Some of the basic differences between Wei and Pi are summarized in Table 8.2:-

Table 8.2 Comparison of Pi and Wei

Wei	Pi
Yang	Yin
Fu	Zang
Hollow	Solid
Receives food & drink	Transforms food & drink
Wei Qi normally descends	Pi Qi normally ascends
Ascent of Wei Qi results in vomiting	Descent of Pi Qi results in diarrhoea
Wei likes Damp, dislikes Dryness	Pi likes Dryness, dislikes Damp
Tends to Deficient Yin, & signs of Heat	Tends to Deficient Yang, & signs of Cold

In practice, certain aspects of Wei and Pi overlap so closely as to be inseparable. Often points from Pi Jing Luo are used for disharmonies of Wei, and points from Wei Jing Luo for disharmonies of Pi.

Functions

Wei is the 'Sea of Grains and Water', the 'Sea of Food and Fluid', responsible for 'receiving' and 'ripening' the food and drink. Transformation of food begins in Wei, the purer faction goes via Pi to Fei, where it becomes Qi, Xue and Jin Ye. The denser, more turbid fraction is sent to Xiao Chang for further digestion and separation of pure from impure. Pi and Wei are complimentary; Pi governs the upward movement of the purer fractions, Wei the descent of the less pure fractions. If the descending power of Wei is disturbed, Wei rebels upward with belching, nausea, and vomiting; and with epigastric pain, discomfort and distention.

Patterns of Disharmony

Retention of Fluid in Wei due to Cold
Retention of Food in Wei
Deficiency of Wei Yin
Blazing Wei Fire

Where Pi tends to Deficiency of Yang and therefore tends to be distressed by Cold and Damp, Wei tends to Deficient Yin and to patterns of Dryness and Heat. However, though Wei does not show the tendency of Pi to invasion by Damp, it does show the tendency to invasion by Cold. In other words, Wei may be associated with patterns of Deficient Yin and Heat and with patterns of Deficient Yang and Cold, depending on the situation. These relationships are summarized in Figure 8.4 below, and are further discussed on pages 203-204.

Figure 8.4 Origins of Wei Disharmony

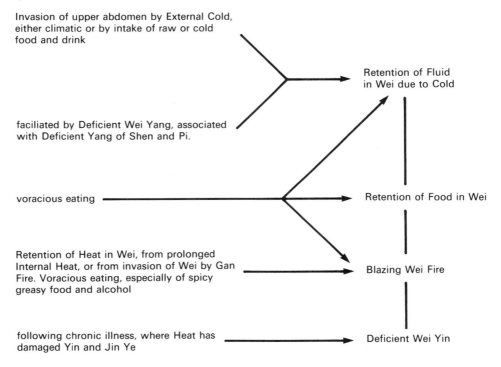

Invasion of upper abdomen by External Cold, either climatic or by intake of raw or cold food and drink

faciliated by Deficient Wei Yang, associated with Deficient Yang of Shen and Pi.

voracious eating

Retention of Heat in Wei, from prolonged Internal Heat, or from invasion of Wei by Gan Fire. Voracious eating, especially of spicy greasy food and alcohol

following chronic illness, where Heat has damaged Yin and Jin Ye

Retention of Fluid in Wei due to Cold

Retention of Food in Wei

Blazing Wei Fire

Deficient Wei Yin

Retention of Fluid in Wei due to Cold

Signs
Coldness and pain in epigastric region, aggravated by cold and alleviated by warmth. Absence of thirst, vomiting after eating, vomiting clear fluid, epigastric sounds, pulse deep and weak, tongue pale with moist or greasy white coat.

Pathology
Accumulation of Cold in Wei, results in Stagnation of Qi and thus in pain. Cold may injure Wei Yang, resulting in absence of thirst. Rebellion of Wei Qi upwards may result in vomiting of clear fluid, which is retained in the stomach, due to Cold damaging the Wei Yang and Pi Yang needed to Transform and to Transport the food and drink. The gurgling sounds in the epigastric region are due to movement of this retained fluid. The pulse is slow due to Cold, and may be weak due to Cold affecting Wei Yang and Pi Yang. The tongue is pale due to depression of Wei and Pi function, with a white coat due to Cold, which is moist or greasy due to accumulation of fluids in Wei.

Treatment

The principle of treatment is to warm and strengthen the Middle Jiao to disperse the Cold and to Transform and Transport the fluid. Reinforcing method and moxa are used. For example, in gastroptosis associated with retention of fluid in Wei due to Cold, the following points may be used:-

Zhongwan	Ren 12 ⎱	This combination of Mu and Shu points for
Weishu	BL.21 ⎰	Wei can regulate Wei Qi, warm the Middle Jiao, and disperse Cold.
Liangmen	ST.21 ⎱	Regulate Wei Qi, and aid gastralgia and
Zusanli	ST.36 ⎰	vomiting.
Quihai	Ren 6	Combined with Zhongwan, warms and invigorates Qi and Yang, and disperses Cold.

Retention of Food in Wei

Signs

Loss of appetite, distension and pain in epigastric region, foul belching and sour regurgitation, loose stool or constipation, foul stool, slippery pulse, and tongue with thick greasy coat.

Pathology

Wei Qi is obstructed and the Wei functions of receiving, storing and digesting food are impaired, with loss of appetite, and distension and pain in the epigastric regions. The retained food may become rotten, so that if Wei Qi rebels, there is belching or regurgitation, which are foul and sour respectively. Also, stool becomes foul, and movement of stool may be impaired, with diarrhoea or constipation, depending on the situation. The slippery pulse and greasy tongue reflect retention of Phlegm and Damp.

Treatment

The principle of treatment is to invigorate the Middle Jiao to aid digestion of food, and remove retention. Reducing or even method are used with points such as the following:-

Xiawan	Ren 10	Enables Wei Qi to go downwards.
Zhangmen	LIV.13	The alarm point of Pi, invigorates Pi to digest food.
Zusanli	ST.36	Dominates ascending of Pi and descending of Wei.

Deficient Wei Yin

Signs

Lack of appetite, dry mouth and lips, dry vomit, constipation, thin rapid pulse, red tongue with no coat.

Pathology
Signs of Deficient Yin, for example constipation, thin rapid pulse, red tongue with no coat, are accompanied by signs of reduced Jin Ye in Wei, and in the mouth and lips which are ruled by Pi. Lack of appetite is a sign of Deficient Wei and Pi.

Treatment
The principle of treatment is to nourish Wei Yin, using reinforcing method and no moxa. Points such as Zusanli, ST.36, Pishu, BL.20, and Weishu, BL.21, may be used to strengthen Wei and Pi functions; and points such as Sanyinjiao, SP.6, and Taixi, KID.3, may be used to strengthen Wei Yin, and Yin in general. This pattern may be found in certain conditions of anxiety and weakness, accompanied by such Yin Deficient signs as emaciation, restlessness, nervousness, insomnia, and sore throat; and by epigastric pain.

Blazing Wei Fire

Signs
Burning pain in epigastrium, thirst with preference for cold drinks, vomiting undigested food or sour fluid. There may be swelling, pain, ulceration and bleeding of the gums; foul breath and constipation. The pulse may be flooding rapid and slippery; and the tongue red with dry thick yellow coat.

Pathology
The majority of these signs are due to Heat. Fire in Wei may blaze upward through Wei Jing Luo to reach the gums, with inflammation and bleeding, and may cause the Wei Qi to ascend with vomiting, and may damage Jin Ye, causing thirst and constipation. The internal Heat manifests as a rapid flooding pulse, and a red tongue with yellow coat. A slippery pulse, and a thick tongue coat may result if the Heat is associated with Damp.

Treatment
Neiting, ST.44, is used to remove Heat, Excess and pain from Wei. Zhongwan, Ren 12, is used to regulate rebellious Wei Qi, and Taichong, LIV.3, is used to pacify Gan and Gan Fire, where present. Liangmen, ST.21, regulates Wei and Pi and is used for epigastric pain, especially when the pain is more lateral. Reducing method is used, as for example in treatment of peptic ulceration associated with Blazing Wei Fire.

Other Wei Disharmonies

Some texts mention further Wei disharmonies. Invasion of Wei by Gan is a progression of Depression of Gan Qi, and may be closely associated with the pattern of Retention of food in Wei, above; hence the sour regurgitation, a Gan sign. This situation is discussed on page 106, as is Invasion of Pi by Gan. Differentiation as to whether the invasion is predominantly of Wei or of Pi will be according to whether the impairment is predominantly of Wei function of descending, vomiting and belching, or predominantly of the Pi function of ascending, with diarrhoea, borborygmus and flatulence.

Some texts include the category of Stagnant Xue in Wei with stabbing, piercing pain, characteristic of Stagnant Xue, in the epigastrium and perhaps radiating around to the back. The pain is aggravated by touch and by eating, since this is an Excess condition. The patient is emaciated with darkish face, and may suffer periodic haematemesis and melaena. The pulse is choppy and wiry, and the tongue is darkish purple with red dots on the sides, and perhaps a thin yellow coat. This pattern may be associated with Heat, that causes the blood vessels to rupture, with the coagulated Xue obstructing the Middle Jiao, causing acute pain. The pattern may be present in certain types of acute or periodic perforation of peptic ulcers.

Summary

Wei patterns may be of Deficiency, for example Deficient Wei Yin; or of Excess, for example Blazing Wei Fire, Retention of Food in Wei, Stagnant Xue in Wei; or of Deficiency turning into Excess, for example Retention of Food in Wei, when this last pattern is precipitated by Deficient Wei Qi and Deficient Pi Qi.

The pattern of Retention of Fluid in Wei due to Cold may be associated with Invasion of Pi by Cold and Damp, and with an underlying Deficiency of Shen, Wei and Pi Yang. Retention of food in Wei may be associated with Depression of Gan Qi; with Cold, as in Retention of Fluid in Wei due to Cold; or with Heat, as in Blazing Wei Fire. The last pattern may be associated with Deficient Wei Yin and Deficient Shen Yin, Blazing Gan Fire, Damp Heat in Gan and Dan, or with Accumulation of Damp Heat in Pi.

The three main Zang Fu involved in these pathological interrelationships are Wei, Pi and Gan, as discussed on page 204.

Table 8.2 Wei Patterns of Disharmony

Pattern	Signs	Pulse	Tongue
Retention of Fluid in Wei due to Cold	coldness & pain in epigastrium, aggravated by cold; vomiting clear fluid	slow weak	moist or greasy white coat
Retention of Food in Wei	distension & pain in epigastrium; sour re-gurgitation; foul belching	slippery	thick greasy coat
Deficient Wei Yin	dry mouth & lips; dry vomit; malar flush; restlessness, anxiety, insomnia	thin rapid	red; no coat
Blazing Wei Fire	burning pain in epigastrium; thirst for cold drink; swollen, painful gums; foul breath; constipation	flooding fast	red; thick dry yellow coat

Chapter
9

Gan (Liver) and Dan (Gall Bladder)

Gan
Functions

1. Rules Free-flowing of Qi
2. Stores Xue
3. Rules the Tendons
4. Opens into the Eyes; Manifests in the Nails

Rules Free-flowing of Qi

This is the most important Gan function. Failure of this function forms the basis of Gan pathology, and is associated with many of the characteristic signs of Gan disharmony.

In simple terms, Pi rules the formation, and hence the quantity, of Post- natal Qi; Fei and Xin govern the movement of Qi throughout the Body, and Gan rules the evenness of that movement.

Gan does not rule the volume or the force of movement of Qi, and is not primarily associated with patterns of Qi Deficiency. Gan rules the evenness of Qi flow; the smooth, unobstructed movement of the Substances throughout the Body, and hence the harmony and regularity of Body functions and of behaviour.

Gan disharmony results in obstruction, blockage and stagnation in the flow of Qi and Substances, and in uneven, irregular and disharmonious function and behaviour.

There are four main facets of the Free-flowing function of Gan:-

Harmony of Emotions
Harmony of Digestion
Secretion of Bile
Harmony of Menstruation

Harmony of Emotions

Gan governs not only the smooth functioning of the Body, but also the harmonious interaction of the individual with the external environment. If the movement of Qi, and the flow of the emotions, is uneven or obstructed, the individual may give inadequate, excessive or inappropriate reactions to environmental stimuli, resulting in disharmonious behaviour, and in disharmony between individual and environment. This involves the common association of the intellectual faculties of planning and decision-making with Gan and Dan respectively.

Harmony of Digestion

The Gan function of Free-flowing of Qi is necessary for the activity of Pi and Wei in digestion. Also, if Gan is disharmonious, stagnant Gan Qi may overflow horizontally into Pi and Wei. This is called Gan Invading Pi and Wei, and results in various digestive disturbances.

Secretion of Bile

The Gan function of Free-flowing of Qi is also involved in the even harmonious secretion of bile. If there is disharmony of this Gan function, secretion of bile is disturbed.

Harmony of Menstruation

The Free-flowing function of Gan is also important in menstruation, where there must be even, unobstructed flow of Qi and Xue. This is related to the second function of Gan, storage of Xue.

Stores Xue

Gan stores Xue, and regulates the quantity of Xue in circulation at any given time. When the Body is active, Xue moves out of Gan into circulation, and when the Body is at rest, Xue returns to Gan. Disharmony of this Gan function may result in too little or too much Xue in circulation, or in irregular fluctuations in the volume of circulating Xue. The interrelationships of Xue with Gan and other Zang Fu are discussed on page 189.

Rules the Tendons

The Chinese term Jin is often translated as Tendons, but may refer to the tendons, ligaments and muscles of Western medicine. Hence the word Tendons is given a capital letter in this book, when referring to the Chinese concept, since it does not exactly correspond to the tendons of Western terminology.

The Tendons, associated with Gan function, refer more to the contractile aspect of muscle function, whereas the Muscles, associated with Pi function, refer more to their bulk and strength. If Gan Xue is Deficient, the Tendons are not properly moistened and nourished by Xue, and their contraction will be impaired and inharmonious, resulting in stiffness, spasms, tremors and numbness. The interrelations of Muscles and Tendons are further discussed on pages 173-4.

Opens into the Eyes; Manifests in the Nails

All the Zang Fu are involved in the proper function of the eyes, and various Zang Fu disharmonies manifest in the eyes. Traditionally, Gan Qi is associated with the ability of the eyes to distinguish the Five Colours, and Gan Xue is associated with good vision. Various Gan disharmony patterns affect the eyes:-

Deficient Gan Xue	blurred vision, dry eyes
Blazing Gan Fire	eyes red, sore, irritated
Stirring of Gan Wind	tremor of eyeball

The interrelationship of eyes with the various Zang Fu is discussed further on page 176.

If Gan stores and regulates Xue properly, the nails are pink and well- formed. Gan disharmonies may result in pale, thin, brittle, ridged nails.

Patterns of Disharmony

Depression of Gan Qi
Deficient Gan Xue
Hyperactive Gan Yang
Blazing Gan Fire
Stirring of Gan Wind
Damp Heat in Gan and Dan
Stagnation of Cold in Gan Jing Luo

The foundations of Gan pathology are:-

1. Depression of Free-flowing of Gan Qi, resulting in Stagnation of Qi and Xue; and in disharmony of digestion, menstruation, emotions and behaviour.
2. Deficiency and irregularity of Gan Xue, resulting in problems of tendons, nails, eyes, and menstruation.
3. Tendency of Gan to Deficiency of Yin, to Dryness and Heat, to Hyperactive Yang and Blazing Fire.
4. Stirring of Gan Wind, due to Deficient Gan Xue, Hyperactive Gan Yang and Blazing Gan Fire, or to severe fever.
5. The combination of Internal or External Damp and Heat, with the tendency of Gan to Stagnation, is associated with the accumulation of Damp Heat in Gan and Dan.
6. The combination of Stagnation due to Depression of Free-flowing of Qi with the Stagnation of Cold, results in Stagnation due to Cold in Gan Jing Luo.

Origins
Figure 9.1 outlines the main origins and interrelationships of the Gan Patterns of Disharmony. The origins of each individual Pattern of Disharmony are discussed below in the appropriate section.

Figure 9.1 Origins of Gan Disharmony

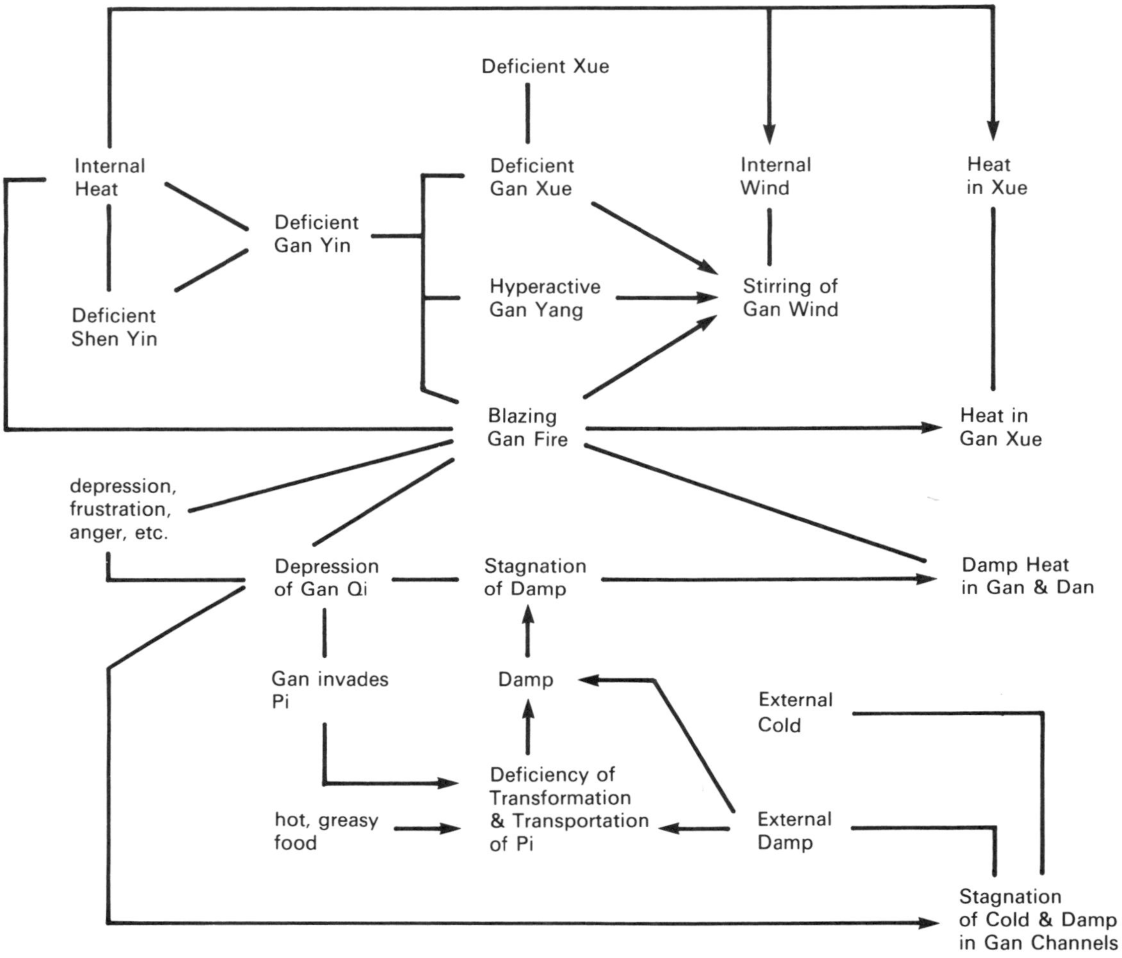

General Gan Signs

Signs of Gan disharmony derive from disharmony of:-

1. Gan functions, for example Free-flowing of Qi as it affects digestion, emotion and menstruation; and storage and regulation of Xue.
2. Tissues and Orifices ruled by Gan, that is Tendons, nails and eyes.
3. Distribution and interconnections of Gan Jing Luo, for example Gan Jing Luo passes through and connects with the head, eyes, hypochondriac and genital regions.

Hence, signs common to all Gan Patterns of Disharmony tend to include digestive disorders, emotional disharmonies, menstrual problems, affections of the tendons, eyes, and head, and distension of the hypochondrium.

Depression of Gan Qi

Origins

This is one of the commonest patterns in clinical practice. Its usual origin is in emotional disharmony, especially depression, frustration, irritability and anger. The relationship between emotional disharmony and Depression of Gan Qi is not so much one of cause and effect, but of mutual interaction:-

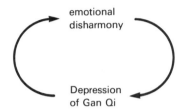

Signs manifested by Depression of Gan Qi include depression, anger, etc.

Signs

The key signs in this pattern are depression, sensation of distension and tenderness of hypochondrium, chest and breasts; poor digestion.

Jing Luo	sensation of distension in hypochondrium in chest, sighing, sensation of 'Plum Seed Qi' in throat, lumps along the Jing Luo
Emotions	depression, frustration, irritation and anger
Digestion	poor appetite, poor digestion, nausea, belching, sour regurgitation and vomiting, epigastric pain, abdominal distension and pain, borborygmus, loose stools
Bile	jaundice, bitter taste, vomiting yellow fluid
Gynaecology	premenstrual signs, for example distension and soreness of lower abdomen and breasts, irritability, etc. Irregular menstruation, amenorrhoea or scanty menstruation, infertility, dysmenorrhoea
Pulse & tongue	pulse wiry; tongue normal or purplish

Pathology

Jing Luo and General

Impairment of Free-flowing of Qi leads to stagnation and accumulation of Qi, and hence to the sensation of distension and pain along the course of the channel. Characteristically, the pain is not severe; it may move in location, and it may come and go, especially with increase and reduction of emotional disturbance. If, however, Stagnation of Qi progresses to Stagnation of Xue, pain is more severe, often stabbing, and does not change location or come and go. The pulse changes from wiry, to wiry and choppy; and the tongue changes from normal, to purplish perhaps with purple spots.

Location of signs depends on the area affected by stagnation. For example, if it is Stagnation of Qi, there may be distension and soreness in the breasts, hypochondrium and abdomen. There may be a stuffy feeling in the chest, accompanied by sighing. The Depression of Gan Qi may invade the throat, combining with Phlegm and cause the foreign body or 'Plum Seed Qi' sensation in the throat, which characteristically comes and goes with depression. Qi and Xue may stagnate at various locations along the course of the channel, forming lumps.

Emotions

Physical, emotional and mental vitality seem stagnant and depressed; and the individual feels low and dispirited. Basic moods of depression may be punctuated by outbursts of anger and irritability.

This pattern emphasises the importance of emotional disturbance in originating disease. Here, depression may precipitate digestive and gynaecological disharmonies, and also pain and discomfort along the course of Gan Jing Luo.

Digestion

There is a very close relationship between Gan and Dan, and Pi and Wei. If depression of Gan Qi invades Pi and Wei, there may be a mixture of Pi and Wei signs. If Gan invades Wei predominantly, Qi tends to ascend, causing nausea, belching, sour regurgitation, vomiting and epigastric pain. If Gan invades predominantly Pi, Qi tends to descend, causing borborygmus, loose stools and abdominal pain.

Bile

If Depression of Gan Qi impairs bile secretion, in addition to general signs of digestive disharmony, for example loss of appetite and nausea, and distension of hypochondria; there may be jaundice, bitter taste and vomiting of yellow fluid.

Gynaecology

In menstruation, Gan communicates with the uterus via Ren Mai and Chong Mai. Gan, Ren Mai and Chong Mai are all concerned with the unobstructed movement of Qi and Xue in menstruation. If there is depression of Gan Qi, there will be an interrupted and uneven flow of Qi and hence of Xue, during menstruation, resulting in irregular and scanty menstruation. There may be sensations of depression and irritability, and of distension and tenderness of abdomen and breasts, which characteristically builds up prior to menstruation and declines once it commences. If the stagnation includes Stagnation of Xue, then dysmenorrhoea will characteristically include severe, stabbing pain, which may be eased by the passing of clots of blood. The interrelationships of Gan and the other Zang Fu in gynaecological disorders are discussed on page 205.

This common pattern of disharmony may exist by itself, may be a precursor for other Gan disharmonies, may co-exist with other Gan disharmonies, may be a precursor of disharmonies of other Zang Fu, for example of Pi and Wei; and may be combined with a variety of syndromes of other Zang Fu.

Treatment
The principle of treatment is to invigorate Gan Qi, and to disperse Stagnation; using even or reducing method. Reducing method is used more in cases of severe pain, as in Stagnant Xue; even method is used more in milder cases with milder pain, as in Stagnant Qi. The points used depend on the combination of disharmonies manifested by the individual, as in the following three examples:-

Premenstrual Tension and Breast Lumps

Taichong	LIV.3	Invigorates Gan, and regulates circulation of Qi and Xue; relieves pain.
Qimen	LIV.14	As above, especially for pain in hyporchondriac and breast region, and as combination with Taichong.
Rugen	ST.18	Specific for breast problems.

Dysmenorrhoea due to Stagnant Xue

Taichong	LIV.3	To disperse Stagnation of Qi and Xue and hence to relieve pain.
Diji	SP.8	Accumulation point of Pi; regulates Xue and uterus, especially for dysmenorrhoea, in combination with Hegu.
Hegu	LI.4	Clears the channels and suppresses pain.

Indigestion and Gastric Pain

Taichong	LIV.3	Regulates Gan to dispel Invasion of Pi and Wei by Gan Qi.
Zhangmen	LIV.13	Regulates Gan Qi, regulates circulation of Qi and Xue, aids Transformation and Transportation by Pi. Alarm point of Pi.
Gongsun	SP.4	Regulates Pi and Wei; relieves pain.

Common Disease Patterns
Depression of Gan Qi may be a component of various diseases:- depression, indigestion, cholecystitis, mastitis, breast lumps, premenstrual tension, amenorrhoea, dysmenorrhoea etc.

Deficiency of Gan Xue

Origins
Factors precipitating Deficient Xue or Gan disharmony, will tend to cause Deficient Gan Xue. For example, loss of blood as in haemorrhages; Deficient formation of Xue as in Deficiency of Pi or of Shen Jing; and injury of Gan, or of Yin and Jin Ye, by Heat, as in febrile diseases or Blazing Gan Fire.

Signs

Face	dull pale
General	emaciation, dizziness
Muscles	weakness, numbness, spasm, tremor
Eyes	dry eyes, blurred vision, spots in visual field
Nails	pale, dry, brittle
Menstruation	amenorrhoea or scanty menses
Pulse & tongue	pulse wiry thin and choppy; tongue pale thin and dry, with little or no coat

The key signs of this pattern are dull pale face, weakness and spasm in Tendons, brittle nails, and scanty menses. The pulse may be wiry, thin, and choppy; and the tongue may be pale and dry.

Pathology

The concept of Gan Xue relates to the storage of Xue, and the regulation of the volume of Xue, by Gan. Deficient Xue means Deficient Gan Xue, and the two patterns share the signs of Deficient Xue, i.e. dull pale complexion, listlessness, numbness or weak tremors in limbs, emaciation and dizziness, thin choppy pulse and pale dry, thin tongue. However, Gan Xue implies a Gan involvement in the disharmony, and includes Gan signs, such as wiry pulse, pale nails, muscle spasms, dry eyes, spots in the visual field, and scanty menses. Nevertheless, the two Patterns of Disharmony greatly overlap, and in clinical practice, Deficient Xue and Deficient Gan Xue are often used almost synonymously.

Treatment

The principle of treatment is to strengthen Xue, and to strengthen the function of Gan to store Xue. Reinforcing method is used, and moxa may be appropriate, providing that there are no signs of Xue Heat.

Deficient Gan Xue is unlikely to be seen in isolation in clinical practice; it is likely to occur with other disharmonies, for example Deficient Gan Yin or general Deficient Xue; in which case, these latter two patterns must also be treated. For example, in a case of spots in the visual field, both Deficient Xue and Deficient Gan Xue occur, and points such as the following may be used:-

Zusanli	ST.36	Strengthen Xue formation by strengthening
Pishu	BL.20	the Transformation function of Pi and Wei.
Taichong	LIV.3	Invigorates Gan function.
Ganshu	BL.18	Strengthens Gan Qi and 'brightens the eyes'.
Guangming	GB.37	Regulates Gan, clears the vision.

Generally, if Deficient Xue and Deficient Gan Xue are accompanied by Deficient Qi signs, moxa is applicable, whereas if they are accompanied by Deficient Yin signs, moxa is not applicable, and points such as Sanyinjiao, SP.6, and Zhaohai, KID.6, may be more appropriate.

Common Disease Patterns

This pattern may be found in such diseases as:- anaemia, nervous exhaustion, hypertension, chronic hepatitis, amenorrhoea, and some chronic eye problems.

Related Disharmonies

Failure of the Gan function to regulate Xue is often associated with Xue Deficiency. However, this failure may also be associated with Depression of Gan Qi, with irregular storage and release of Xue, resulting, for example in irregular, on/off menstruation. Alternatively, failure of the Gan function to regulate Xue may be combined with Xue Heat, resulting in excess Xue in circulation, and in a tendency of Xue to leave the Vessels, as in menorrhagia, and metrorrhagia. This last combination of disharmonies would manifest signs of Heat, whereas haemorrhage due to inability of Pi to hold in Xue within Xue Mai, would manifest signs of Cold and of Deficient Yang.

Stagnation of Xue, due to Depression of Gan Qi or to other causes, may interact with Deficient Gan Xue as follows:—

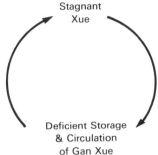

Deficient Gan Xue may result in stirring of Gan Wind, discussed on page 115.

Hyperactive Gan Yang

Origins and Interrelationships

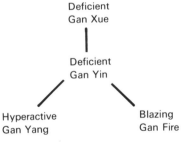

The four Gan patterns, Deficient Gan Xue, Deficient Gan Yin, Hyperactive Gan Yang, and Blazing Gan Fire, are so closely interwoven, that they are often difficult to separate in clinical Practice.

These patterns may be represented as four continua:-

Deficient Gan Yin ——— Deficient Gan Xue
Deficient Gan Yin ——— Hyperactive Gan Yang
Deficient Gan Yin ——— Blazing Gan Fire
Blazing Gan Fire ——— Hyperactive Gan Yang

The central pattern, Deficient Gan Yin, is not listed as a main Gan pattern, it is regarded more as a precursor to, or an accompaniment of, the other three patterns.

Prolonged Internal Heat, Deficient Shen Yin, loss of Xue or Deficient Xue, may develop into Deficient Gan Yin. This may manifest as signs of Deficient Yin in the context of Gan, i.e. general Deficient Yin signs, such as palms and soles hot, afternoon fever, thin rapid pulse, and thin red tongue; plus Gan signs, such as spots in the visual field and wiry pulse.

Deficient Gan Xue and Deficient Gan Yin reflect the underlying relationship of Deficient Xue and Deficient Yin, and their links with Deficient Jin Ye and signs of Dryness and thinness. Deficient Gan Xue and Deficient Gan Yin form a continuum, in which one pattern may predominate at a particular time. The signs of Heat with red tongue and rapid pulse may indicate predominance of Deficient Gan Yin; signs of dull pale face, choppy pulse and pale tongue, may indicate predominance of Deficient Gan Xue.

Deficient Gan Yin, Hyperactive Gan Yan and Blazing Gan Fire may be seen as a continuum starting with Deficient Gan Yin and progressing through Hyperactive Gan Yang to Blazing Gan Fire; with signs increasing in severity from Deficient Gan Yin to Blazing Gan Fire. For example, dizziness or headache may be mild, moderate or severe. However, the differentiation between these three patterns is not just of quantity but also of quality. For example, although Hyperactive Gan Yang must always be associated with Deficient Gan Yin, and therefore tends to show some signs of Heat, the Heat signs are not necessarily more severe than Deficient Gan Yin, indeed they may be less prominent.

In a Deficient Gan Yin - Hyperactive Gan Yang pattern, signs of either Deficient Gan Yin or Hyperactive Gan Yang may predominate; if the former, there may be signs of Deficient Heat and possibly signs common to Deficient Gan Yin and Deficient Gan Xue, for example emaciation, blurred vision and thin pulse, may be emphasized. If Hyperactive Gan Yang predominates, there may be the characteristic distending headache, fewer signs of Deficient Heat, and a pulse which is less thin and more floating.

Though Hyperactive Gan Yang has some signs of Excess, it is based on Deficiency and weakness, and can be differentiated from Blazing Gan Fire by the greater strength of the signs in the case of the latter. For example, where a headache is merely distending and throbbing in the case of Hyperactive Gan Yang, for Blazing Gan Fire it is severe and splitting. In Hyperactive Gan Yan there are small outbursts of moderate anger, and in Blazing Gan Fire there may be violent fits of rage. Also, the Deficient Heat signs in Deficient Gan Yin become Excess Heat signs in Blazing Gan Fire, for example the whole Body is hot and the whole face red, rather than palms and soles hot, with malar flush; and the pulse is full and rapid, not thin and rapid.

This situation becomes more complex, when in addition to the co-existence of the four patterns mentioned above, there is also Depression of Gan Qi, or when one or all of Deficient Gan Xue, Hyperactive Gan Yang and Blazing Gan Fire give rise to Stirring of Gan Wind. Patterns of Damp may also develop from these five syndromes, for example Damp Heat in Gan and Dan; or Pi disharmonies, such as Turbid Phlegm Disturbing the Head, with signs of great dizziness, slippery pulse and thick, greasy tongue. This may occur in some patterns of Wind corresponding to the CVA of Western medicine.

Signs
The signs of this pattern derive from the interaction of the following three aspects:- Deficient Yin, Hyperactive Yang, and Gan.

110

Deficient Gan Yin	palms and soles hot, insomnia, dry eyes, spots in visual field, dizziness, dry mouth
Headache	distending, throbbing headache, especially in temples and/or vertex; tinnitus
Emotions	anger and irritability
Tendons	numbness, spasm, tremor
Pulse & Tongue	pulse wiry and rapid; more floating if Hyperactive Yang predominates, and more thin and rapid if Deficient Gan Yin predominates. Tongue red with little coat, perhaps dry

The key signs of this pattern are anger and irritability; and distending, throbbing, temporal/vertical headache; with some signs of Heat.

Pathology
The basis of such patterns as Hyperactive Gan Yang, Blazing Gan Fire and Stirring of Gan Wind, is that Gan Yin is insufficient to control Gan Yang or Gan Fire, which subsequently rise to the upper part of the Body and the head. The Yang rises, carrying Excess Qi and Xue to the head, with feelings of fullness and distension, especially in areas of the Gan channel, for example, the vertex, and the Dan channel, for example, the temporal area.

Deficient Yin gives rise to sensation of hot palms and soles, dry mouth, thin rapid pulse and red tongue with little coat. Deficient Gan Yin and/or Deficient Gan Xue originate signs of dry eyes, and spots in the visual field. General Gan signs are numbness, spasm and trembling of Muscles and Tendons and wiry pulse.

Dizziness and insomnia can each occur with Deficient Yin, Deficient Xue, Deficient Gan Yin, Deficient Gan Xue and Hyperactive Gan Yang; differentiation would be on the basis of predominant accompanying signs. For example, dizziness and insomnia due to Blazing Gan Fire would be severe and accompanied by other very severe signs.

Treatment
The principle of treatment is to pacify Gan Yang, and to nourish Gan Yin. Reducing or even method is used to pacify Gan Yang, and reinforcing method is used to nourish Gan Yin. Points such as the following may be used:-

Taichong	LIV.3 ⎱	Both points pacify Hyperactive Gan Yang.
Xingjian	LIV.2 ⎰	Taichong is used in more chronic, Xingjian in more acute cases.
		These points are usually used separately, not together
Fengchi	GB.20	Pacifies Yang in the head, and benefits the eyes.
Baihui	Du 20	Pacifies Gan, Yang and mind.

If there is a strong underlying Deficient Yin pattern, points such as Shenshu, BL.23, and Taixi, KID.3, may be added.

Common disease patterns.

This pattern may manifest in cases of:- hypertension, headaches, emotional disturbance, vertigo, tinnitus, premenstrual tension, hyperthyroidism, and in severe progressions, with CVA sequellae.

Blazing Gan Fire

In the balance of Deficient Gan Yin, Hyperactive Gan Yang and Blazing Gan Fire, the predominant pattern will depend upon:-

1. Strength and type of constitution
    A strong constitution tends to signs of fullness, in this case of Excess Heat; a weak constitution tends to signs of Deficiency, in this case Deficient Heat. Generally, in a strong constitution, the signs may be more severe than with a weak constitution, for example the headache is more solid and severe.
2. Circumstances
    A single person may at one time manifest signs of Deficient Gan Yin, for example malar flush and mild sensations of Heat; at another time manifest signs of Hyperactive Gan Yang, with fullness in the head; and on yet another occasion, manifest signs of Blazing Gan Fire with severe headache, redness of the whole face and violent anger. The first situation may be associated with a period of tiredness and exhaustion, the second with a period of moderate stress, and the third with a period of extreme aggravation, frustration and annoyance.

Origins

A past history of Internal Heat and/or Deficient Gan Yin may predispose to Blazing Gan Fire. This pattern may also arise from chronic Depression of Gan Qi; in TCM, Stagnation may eventually, over a period of time, give rise to Heat and flare up as Fire. Severe anger and annoyance, alcohol and tobacco, rich and greasy food may contribute to this pattern.

Signs

Full Fire	thirst, constipation, dark urine, red face red eyes, insomnia, haemorrhage
Head	violent headache, sudden tinnitus or deafness
Emotions	violent anger
Gan invades Pi and Wei	bitter taste, sour regurgitation, nausea, pain in hyperchondrium
Pulse & tongue	pulse wiry rapid and full; tongue red, with thick yellow coat

The key signs in this pattern are violent anger and violent headaches, plus signs of Excess Heat, and full, rapid wiry pulse.

Pathology

Blazing Gan Fire shares with the patterns of general Excess Heat or Blazing Fire, the general Excess Heat signs, for example, red tongue with yellow coat, full rapid pulse, thirst, bitter taste, constipation, etc. These signs arise from the effect of Heat on Yin and Jin Ye, and hence on Shen★. If Xin Yin and Xin Xue are damaged due to extreme Heat affecting Jin Ye, then Shen★ has no Residence, is Disturbed, and insomnia results. The patterns of Blazing Xin Fire and Blazing Gan Fire are often closely associated, and the former may arise from the latter. Blazing Gan Fire is distinguished by the sudden severe signs of anger, headache, tinnitus and deafness; resulting from sudden ascent of hot Qi and Xue to the head, ascending the Gan and Dan channels, with their distributions in the vertex and the temporal regions respectively. Sour regurgitation is often associated with Blazing Gan Fire, especially if Gan invades Pi and Wei. The wiry quality of the pulse is due to Gan, and the full and rapid qualities due to Excess Heat. The red tongue with dry yellow coat, is a result of Excess Heat; and the redness or red spots on the side of the tongue indicate Gan disharmony.

This pattern is the extreme case of failure of the Free-flowing function of Gan Qi resulting in disharmony between the individual and the environment. The individual may be hypersensitive and liable to explode with rage. Sudden outbursts of extreme anger, occasionally involving physical violence, are rarely conducive to the smooth, even flow of social interaction.

Treatment

The principle of treatment is to reduce Gan Fire, using reducing method, and by bleeding certain points. Moxa is contra-indicated. Points such as the following may be used, depending on the particular requirements of the patient:-

Xingjiang	LIV.2	Pacifies acute flare-up of Gan Fire.
Fengchi	GB.20	Pacifies Gan and Yang and Heat in the Head
Zanzhu	BL.2 ⎫	Bleed these points to disperse Heat locally and
Taiyang	M-HN-9 ⎭	pacify mind.
Yongquan	KID.1	May be added to pacify Fire, strengthen Yin and calm Shen★. Indicated for headache at vertex, vertigo, blurred vision and insanity.

Common Disease Patterns

This pattern includes :- hypertension, abnormal uterine bleeding, migraine, acute conjunctivitis and glaucoma, otitis, Menières disease, haemorrhage of upper digestive tract, violent behaviour.

Stirring of Gan Wind

The concept of Wind in Chinese medicine indicates rapid, changing movement. Wind is light and Yang and rises, hence it predominantly affects the upper Body, especially the head. Internal and External Wind share these characteristics, but have very different origins and signs, and do not generally give rise to each other. Internal Wind is largely, though not necessarily, associated with Gan disharmony, since it is sudden, irregular movement, the opposite of the smooth, even flow promoted by Gan. Internal Wind affects the upper Body as Wind affects the upper branches of a tree, producing signs of rapid change of movement, characteristically tics, tremors, spasms and convulsions. The disruptive effect of these rapid, abnormal gusts and squalls of upward movement on the circulation of Qi and Xue, may have drastic consequences within the Body, resulting in dizziness or even loss of consciousness.

Types
There are three main patterns of Stirring of Gan Wind:-

Utmost Heat producing Wind
Deficient Yin and Hyperactive Yang producing Wind
Deficient Xue and Deficient Gan Xue producing Wind

Production of Utmost Heat occurs only in severe febrile diseases. It is a full, sudden, serious, acute condition. This is different from Blazing Gan Fire, arising from Depression of Gan Qi or Deficient Gan Yin, which is more likely to be associated with the second category, that of Wind produced from Deficient Gan Yin and Hyperactive Yang.

Blazing Gan Fire may be Excess based on Deficiency, and although it may be serious, it is more likely to be acute flare-ups arising from a chronic condition of Deficiency, than the sudden, acute, full condition of the first category. Finally, Wind deriving from Deficient Gan Xue is a condition of chronic emptiness, with signs of much lesser severity.

These three patterns share two common factors in the origin of Internal Wind.

1. Deficient Yin and Deficient Xue
In the first category, Yin and Xue are damaged by the extreme Heat. The second category includes Deficiency of Yin, and often also Deficiency of Xue, which may be further aggravated by the Blazing of Gan Fire. The third category is based on Deficient Xue, and is often accompanied by Deficient Yin. Deficient Yin and Deficient Xue result in lack of nourishment and moisture for muscles and tendons, resulting in their weakness, numbness, stiffness and spasticity.

2. Turbulence
The powerful upward rushing Fire of Utmost Heat creates great turbulence in the upward movement of Qi and Xue. Similarly, the strong upward surge of Hyperactive Yang, when uncontrolled by Yin, creates turbulence in its wake. This disruptive, turbulent movement is Internal Wind. Deficient Xue means insufficient Xue to maintain a strong, steady, even flow of Xue through the Jing Luo and Xue Mai, resulting in a weak, fluctuating, uneven flow. This lesser, but more chronic, turbulence is the Internal Wind derived from Deficient Xue.

In a sense, Stirring of Gan Wind is simply a specific and extreme form of the changing uneven movement to which Gan is prone. The combination of the two factors of Deficient Yin and Xue, and turbulence, creates the characteristic signs of Stirring of Gan Wind.

Origins
Origins of Stirring of Gan Wind have been discussed, and are outlined in Figure 9.1. Internal Wind may also arise from Phlegm and Heat, formed by eating excess sweet or fatty foods and alcohol.

Signs
Generally the main signs of Stirring of Gan Wind are:- tics, tremors, convulsions, numbness, spasms, dizziness and sometimes loss of consciousness.

Specific signs of the three different types of Stirring of Gan Wind are outlined in Table 9.1 below.

Pathology

Utmost Heat
The extreme turbulence and Heat caused by the violent upward movement of Fire and Yang, is so disruptive to the flow of Qi and Xue, that it results in extreme and uncontrolled movement and contraction of Muscles and Tendons; with convulsions, neck spasms and opisthotonos. The extreme Heat injures Shen*, with coma and delirium.

Hyperactive Yang
There may be signs due to Deficient Gan Yin, Hyperactive Yang and Blazing Gan Fire, but the most important are signs due to the turbulence caused by the uprush of Yang; this results in disturbance of Xin and Brain, Shen* and Senses, and thus in loss of consciousness or mental disorientation, with possible impairment of speech. If turbulent Yang and Fire invade Jing Luo of the upper Body, they may disrupt the flow of Qi and Xue, with hemiplegia or facial paralysis.

Table 9.1 Comparison of the Signs of the Three Types of Internal Wind

Signs	Utmost Heat	Hyperactive Yang	Deficient Xue
Heat signs	severe, high fever	none, or relatively mild	usually none
Tendons	convulsions, rigidity, opisthotonos	hemiplegia	numbness, trembling, spasm of head and extremities
Senses	coma, delirium	sudden loss of consciousness, mental disorder, aphasia	blurring of vision, dizziness
Pulse	wiry, rapid, full	wiry, perhaps rapid, thin	wiry, choppy, thin
Tongue	scarlect; dry yellow coat	red; dry variable coat	pale, dry; no coat

Deficient Xue
There may be signs of Deficient Xue and Deficient Gan Xue; otherwise the only additional signs in this case of Stirring of Gan Wind is emphasis on trembling and convulsion, for reasons stated.

Phlegm and Wind

Phlegm and Fire are often associated in pathology, and Fire may give rise to Wind, so that Wind and Phlegm may occur together.

Extreme Heat can cause loss of consciousness by Disturbance of Shen*; and Wind and Phlegm can also cause loss of consciousness by disruption and obstruction respectively, of the circulation of Qi and Xue in Jing Luo of the head, thus clouding the Orifices of the Senses. Phlegm may also obstruct the Orifices of Xin, causing disturbance and obstruction of Shen*.

Wind and Phlegm may occur together, as in Penetrating Wind or in seizures, which roughly correspond to the CVA and epilepsy of Western medicine, respectively. In both cases, the Wind and Phlegm rebel upward, disrupting the flow of Qi in the channels so that circulation of Qi in the head becomes disorderly. Hence, the Orifices of the Senses become disconnected, so that the ears do not hear properly, and the eyes do not see properly, and there may be dizziness and collapse.

The turbulence and obstruction due to Wind and Phlegm may also affect the Jing Luo resulting in the paralysis, and especially hemiplegia, typical of CVA sequellae.

Treatment

Utmost Heat

The principle of treatment is to reduce Heat and to pacify Gan Wind, using reducing method and the bleeding of certain points. Moxa is obviously contra-indicated. Points such as the following may be used:-

Fengchi	GB.20	Pacify Yang, Fire and Wind of Gan, and calm the mind.
Taichong	LIV.3	
Fengfu	Du 16	Fengfu pacifies Wind, and Dazhui clears Heat. Both clear the Brain and calm Shen*, and relieve muscle spasm.
Dazhui	Du 14	
Hegu	LI.4	Hegu, especially in combination with Dazhui, clears Heat, and thus relieves muscle spasm.
Shixuan	M-UE-1	Bleed to clear Heat and restore consciousness.

Du Mai is called the 'Governing Channel', or the 'Sea of Yang Channel', since it controls all the Yang channels. Being the topmost part of the Body, the meeting place of all the Yang channels, and because Yang rises, the head and the Du channel are especially prone to excess or to turbulence of Yang, as in the conditions of Hyperactive Yang, Blazing Fire, extreme Heat, or Internal Wind. Du Mai has links with the Brain, and with the Orifices of the Senses. Thus Excess or turbulence of Yang may result in loss of consciousness, and the extreme Heat associated with febrile conditions may cause severe spasm of Muscles and Tendons and convulsions. This explains the use of Fengfu and Dazhui above to regulate Yang and to disperse Excess from Du Mai.

Hyperactive Yang

Various disease patterns are associated with Deficient Yin, Hyperactive Yang, Blazing Fire and Stirring of Gan Wind. For example, Windstroke and epilepsy.

The principle of treatment and the points used will depend on the particular pattern and the particular patient involved.

For example, Windstroke is divided into:-

1. Acute pattern, associated with Zang Fu involvement, subdivided into 'closed' and 'abandoned' types.
2. Pattern of sequellae of Windstroke, associated with Jing Luo involvement.

The principle of treatment in the closed pattern is to clear the Orifices, drain Heat, and pacify Rebellious Qi. The principle of treatment in the abandoned pattern aims at stabilising Yang. The principle of treatment in sequellae of stroke is to clear Jing Luo, invigorate circulation of Qi and Xue, and eliminate Wind. Reducing method is used in the closed type, reinforcing method in the abandoned type. In later stages, after closed type has progressed to abandoned type, moxa is appropriate. For sequellae of stroke, points may be chosen according to area or function affected, for example arm, leg, speech; and even method and moxa are used. For details of points, see references 9 & 18.

In epilepsy, or seizures, the principle of treatment is to clear the Orifices of the head, i.e. of the Senses, transform Phlegm and pacify Gan Wind. During a seizure, reducing method is used; between seizures, even method is used. Points may be selected from such as the following:-

Yongquan	KID.1	Calms Shen*, opens the Orifices of the Senses.
Yaoqi	M-BW-29	Specific point for epileptic seizures.
Fengchi	GB.20	
Fengfu	Du 16	Pacify Wind, calm Shen*, clear the Brain.
Dazhui	Du 14	
Renzhong	Du 26	Regulates Yin and Yang, opens the Orifices of the head to restore consciousness.

Various other points could also be added, depending on the situation, for example, on whether the seizures are mainly in the night or in the day, whether it is grand or petit mal; and also points may be added to clear Phlegm, to relax Muscles and Tendons, to Strengthen Yin, etc.

Deficient Xue

For example, tic of eye, or tremor of head. The principle of treatment is to pacify Wind, using even method, and to nourish Xue using reinforcing method. Points may be selected from such as the following;-

Taichong	LIV.3	
Fengchi	GB.20	Pacify Gan and disperse Wind, especially in the Head
Baihui	Du 20	
Hegu	LI.4	Disperses Wind and clears the channels.
Zusanli	ST.36	Strengthen the function of Pi and Wei to form Xue
Pishu	BL.20	
Ganshu	BL.18	Strengthens Gan Xue.
Geshu	BL.17	Strengthens Xue.

Common Disease Patterns
Examples of Common Disease Patterns in which the Stirring of Gan Wind is involved are:-

Extreme Heat	febrile disease, for example encephalitis B
Hyperactive Yang	CVA and sequellae, epilepsy
Deficient Xue	tics and tremors, especially of eyes and head

Damp Heat in Gan and Dan

Origins
The origins of this pattern are summarised in Figure 9.1. If Transformation and Transportation function of Pi is impaired, for example by external Damp or by Invasion by Gan, Internal Damp may be produced. If there is Depression of Gan Qi, the Damp may Stagnate, producing Heat. This pattern is aggravated by consumption of rich, greasy food, alcohol etc.

Signs
The main signs of this pattern are associated with Depression of Gan Qi, Heat and Damp, and Invasion of Pi by Gan.

Depression of Gan Qi	sensations of fullness and pain in chest and hypochondrium, jaundice, bitter taste
Gan Invades Pi	loss of appetite, nausea, vomiting sour, abdominal distension
Heat	fever, thirst, dark urine
Pulse and Tongue	pulse is wiry rapid and slippery; tongue is red with greasy yellow coat

The red tongue with greasy coat, and slippery rapid pulse distinguish this pattern from other Gan disharmonies.

Pathology
The pathology of the signs of Depression of Gan Qi, impaired secretion of bile, and Invasion of Pi by Gan, have been discussed. The red tongue, rapid pulse, fever etc., arise from Internal Heat; the Damp in the system, which may congeal to form Phlegm, produces the slippery pulse and greasy tongue coat.

Treatment
For example, in leucorrhoea of the Damp Heat type, the principle of treatment is to regulate Dai Mai, Chong Mai and Ren Mai; and to disperse Damp Heat. Reducing or even method is used, and points such as the following may be selected:-

Daimai	GB.26	Strengthens Dai Mai and helps to eliminate Damp Heat and therefore discharge.
Qihai	Ren 6	Invigorates Qi circulation, reduces Stagnation and accumulation of Damp.
Sanyinjiao	SP.6	Strengthens Pi to eliminate Damp.

Yinlingquan	SP.9	Strengthens Pi to eliminate Damp Heat.
Zhongji	Ren 3 ⎫	Zhongji is the Crossing point of Ren and Gan
Ligou	LIV.5 ⎭	channels, and Ligou is the Luo point of the Gan channel. In combination, these points reduce Fire of Gan, and clear the channels and alleviate Damp Heat.

For example in cholecystitis, the principle of treatment is to spread and drain Dan Qi, eliminate Damp Heat, invigorate the Middle Jiao and calm Wei. The method of treatment, during the attack of pain, is to needle Dannangxue and Neiguan with reducing method until the pain is relieved. Then, the other points are used with even method.

Dannangxue	M-LE-23	Specific point for Dan disharmony.
Neiguan	P.6	Expands Middle Jiao and harmonises Wei.
Yanglingquan	GB.34 ⎫	Spread and drain Dan Qi.
Riyue	GB.24 ⎭	
Sanyinjiao	SP.6 ⎫	Strengthen Pi to eliminate Damp Heat.
Yinglingquan	SP.9 ⎭	
Zusanli	ST.36	Strengthens Pi and Wei and Middle Jiao.

Common Disease Patterns
Damp Heat in Gan and Dan may be associated with the Western categories of jaundice, hepatitis, cholelethaisis, cholecystitis, and leucorrhoea.

Stagnation of Cold in Gan Jing Luo

Origins
Both Internal and External Cold, and Depression of Gan Qi may contribute to this pattern, since these may all lead to Stagnation of Qi in Gan Jing Luo.

Signs
Pain and distension in lower abdomen, testes and scrotum, alleviated by warmth. Pulse wiry deep and slow. Tongue pale with white coat.

Pathology
Since Cold concentrates in the lower part of the Body, and since Gan Jing Luo surrounds the genitals, pain and swelling may be especially in these areas. Cold is also characterised by contraction, and by obstruction of Qi, accompanied by pain. Cold results in the deep, slow pulse and pale tongue with white coat. A wiry or tight pulse may result from the combination of pain and Cold.

Treatment
The principle of treatment is to invigorate circulation of Qi to disperse Cold, and to clear Gan Jing Luo. Even method of manipulation is used, with moxa.

Ligou	LIV.5 ⎫	Combined to clear Gan Jing Luo and reduce pain in testes.
Taichong	LIV.3 ⎭	
Qihai	Ren 6	Moxa, to invigorate Qi and Yang, and to disperse
Guanyuan	Ren 4	Cold from Lower Jiao.

Table 9.2 Gan Patterns of Disharmony

Pattern	Signs	Pulse	Tongue
Depression of Gan Qi	depression; sensations of distension or tenderness of hypochondrium, chest and breasts; menstrual and digestive disturbances	wiry ± white	normal or purplish; greasy coat
Deficient Gan Xue	dull pale face; weakness and spasm in Tendons and Muscles; dry nails; scanty menses	wiry thin choppy	pale & dry
Hyperactive Gan Yang	irritability and anger; distending headache, especially in temples and vertex; dry mouth	wiry thin sl. rapid	red, dry; little coat
Blazing Gan Fire	violent anger; violent headache; whole face red; thirst; bitter taste	wiry full rapid	red, dry; thick yellow coat
Stirring of Gan Wind (Utmost Heat)	high fever; coma; neck rigidity; opisthotonos	wiry thin rapid	scarlet, dry; yellow coat
Stirring of Gan Wind (Hyperactive Yang)	sudden syncope; speech difficulties; hemiplegia	wiry thin ± rapid	red, dry
Stirring of Gan Wind (Deficient Xue)	sallow face; blurred vision; dizziness; tremor, numbness or spasm of upper extremities	wiry thin	pale, dry
Damp Heat in Gan and Dan	pain in hypochondrium; jaundice; nausea; bitter taste ± fever	wiry slippery rapid	red; greasy yellow coat
Stagnation of Cold in Gan Jing Luo	pain and distension in lower abdomen and testes; alleviated by warmth	deep wiry slow	pale, moist; white coat

Summary

The most important Gan function is governing the Free-flowing of Qi. Failure of this function may result in Depression of Gan Qi, Stagnation of Qi, and Stagnation of Xue; irregularity and stagnation of the flow of bile, the emotions, and the menstrual cycle; and Invasion of Pi and Wei by Gan, with attendant digestive problems. Also, stagnation may lead to Heat and Fire, and to Damp Heat and Phlegm Fire. In other circumstances, stagnation may be associated with the accumulation of Cold and Damp in Gan Jing Luo.

Gan needs moisture and is prone to Deficient Yin, and to Hyperactive Yang and Blazing Fire. Failure of the Gan function of Storing Xue may lead to Deficient Gan Xue, manifesting in face, lips, tongue, pulse, Tendons, eyes, nails, menstrual cycle, etc. Failure of this function may also lead to irregularity in the storage and release of Xue by Gan, associated with haemorrhage, especially if aggravated by Heat in Xue.

Extreme Heat, Deficient Gan Yin accompanied by Hyperactive Gan Yang and Blazing Fire, or Deficient Gan Xue, may all be accompanied by Stirring of Gan Wind; the extreme form of the irregular movement of Qi and Xue manifested by Gan.

Dan

Functions

Gan produces bile and Dan stores it, releasing it periodically so that it moves downward to Xiao Chang to aid digestion. Dan is listed as a Curious Organ, because it resembles a Yang organ system in form, since it is hollow, yet resembles a Yin organ system in function, since it stores a pure fluid, bile. It is unlike the other Fu systems, all of which are involved in the process of receiving and transforming food and drink, and eliminating waste.

Gan and Dan are so closely linked that it is very difficult to separate their functions and disharmonies, and those of Dan are often included in those of the dominant partner, Gan. For example, if disharmony of Gan is associated with irregular supply of bile, this will affect Dan; and if disharmony of Dan is associated with disorder of the healthy rhythm of storage and release of bile, this may affect Gan.

Hence, the two systems are often both involved in such disorders as jaundice, hepatitis, cholecystitis, cholelithiasis, and digestive disorders including vomiting of sour material. Points from both Gan and Dan channels may be used.

Gan and Dan are also closely linked in their emotional and intellectual aspects. Both are characterised by anger and irritability. Where Gan is responsible for proper planning, Dan is responsible for making decisions and judgements. Deficiency or disharmony of Dan may be accompanied by indecision and timidity. The fearfulness sometimes associated with Dan disharmony tends to be associated with indecision, whereas the fearfulness associated with Xin disharmony tends to be associated with feelings of panic and anxiety. However, both Xin and Dan disharmonies may be accompanied by restlessness and irritability, so differentiation between the two patterns must be based on other criteria.

Patterns of Disharmony

Disharmonies of Dan are generally included in disharmonies of Gan, for example Damp Heat in Gan and Dan. However, there is the relatively minor Dan disharmony variously called **Deficient Dan Heat** and **Deficient Dan Qi**. The pattern sometimes termed **Excess Dan Heat** has very similar signs to the pattern of Damp Heat in Gan and Dan, and has not been listed separately in Table 9.3

Table 9.3 Dan Patterns of Disharmony

Pattern	Signs	Pulse	Tongue
Damp Heat in Gan and Dan	pain in hypochondrium; jaundice; nausea; bitter taste; ±fever	wiry slippery rapid	red; greasy yellow coat
Deficient Dan Qi	indecision, timidity, fearfulness, irritability; vertigo; blurred vision	wiry thin	thin white coat

Chapter
10

Xin (Heart) and Xiao Chang (Small Intestine)

Xin

Functions

1. Rules Xue and Xue Mai
2. Stores Shen*
3. Opens into the Tongue; Manifests in the Face

The main functions of Xin are that it rules Xue and Xue Mai, and stores Shen*.

The relatively more Yang function of Xin, the movement of Xue within Xue Mai, is closely related to the relatively Yin function of Xin, that of storing, or of providing a Residence for Shen*. This interrelationship is shown in Figure 10.1.

Figure 10.1 Yin Yang Relationships of Xin

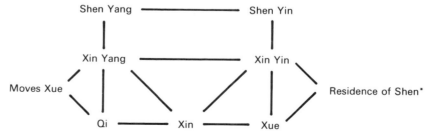

Of course Figure 10.1 is an oversimplification, since, for example, Deficient Xin Qi and Deficient Xin Xue may occur together, and may be associated with Deficient Xin Yin or Deficient Xin Yang.

Rules Xue and Xue Mai

The relationship between Xue, Xue Mai, Mai and Qi has been discussed on page 9, and may be represented by Figure 10.2.

Zong Qi, the Qi of the chest, aids the movement of Xin in the heartbeat, and the movement of Fei in respiration. It also assists Xin in the movement of Xue, and Fei in the movement of Qi, through the channel network, and through the Tissues of the Body.

Figure 10.2 Xin Relationships

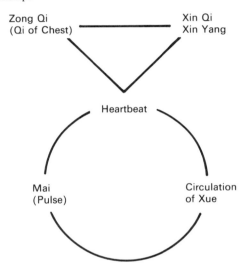

Qi moves Xue, and Fei rules Qi; Xue nourishes Qi, and Xin regulates the movement of Xue. There is a very close relationship between Qi and Xue, Xin and Fei, and Zong Qi. Within Xin itself, Xin Qi and Xin Xue are mutually dependent, and must be abundant and harmoniously balanced for heartbeat and pulse to be even and normal. Also, the state of Xue Mai depends on the harmony of Xin and Xue; traditionally, Xue Mai is the Tissue governed by Xin.

Xue and Xue Mai do not exactly correspond to the Western concept of blood and blood vessels. TCM has little interest in the detailed composition of Xue and Xue Mai; it is concerned with their physiology, and especially with their pathology. Also, the distinction between Qi and Xue, Jing Luo and Xue Mai is often blurred. This is especially so in the case of Ying Qi, which closely resembles Xue, and which flows with it in Jing Luo and Xue Mai.

Stores Shen★

Xin rules Shen★. In TCM, Xin is said to store Shen★; Xin is the Residence of Shen★. Hence, in TCM, Xin is the seat of consciousness, rather than the brain, as in Western medicine.

Xin requires adequate Xin Xue and Xin Yin to house Shen★ properly. If either or both of these are Deficient, Shen★ has no Residence, and becomes Disturbed. If Shen★ is harmonious, the mind is calm and peaceful, and there is clear consciousness and mental activity. If Shen★ is Disturbed, the mind is restless, with insomnia, confused thinking, poor memory, or even loss of consciousness.

Gan and Xin are the two Zang Fu most closely concerned with maintaining a harmonious balance of the emotion; and a smooth, adequate and appropriate flow of reactions to environmental stimuli. If Shen★ is Disturbed, there may be feelings of restlessness, anxiety and panic. In severe cases there may be confused, irrational, manic or hysterical behaviour; and insanity, delirium and loss of consciousness. If Shen★ is Deficient, the individual may feel joyless, lifeless, apathetic and dull. If Shen★ is Deficient, or especially if Shen★ is Disturbed, the individual's emotions and behavioural responses are no longer appropriate, leading to further environmental disharmony. For example, manic and hysterical behaviour are likely to cause difficulty in human relationships, and hence further problems for the patient.

There is a close relationship between Deficient Yin, Deficient Xue, Disturbance of Shen★, and emotional disharmony. Deficient Yin and Deficient Xue may originate, or be originated by, emotional disharmony. Similarly, Disturbance of Shen★ may give rise to emotional disharmony, or, may be originated by it, either directly or via the chronic conditions of Deficient Yin and Deficient Xue. For example, insomnia may give rise to Deficient Yin and Deficient Xue, and hence to Disturbance of Shen★. Alternatively, Disturbance of Shen★, as in Blazing Xin Fire, may give rise to restlessness and insomnia.

As discussed on page 12, the word Shen★ has been used in preference to Spirit, since in Western understanding spirit implies the opposite of matter, animating it, but separate from it. In TCM, Shen★ has its material aspect, it is the manifestation of the activity of Jing and Qi, and is not separable from the functions of Xin and Xue.

Manifests in the Face; Opens into the Tongue
The complexion reflects, among other things, the state of Xin and Xue. If Xin and Xue are abundant, complexion is rosy and bright. If Xin and Xue are Deficient, the complexion is pale and dull.

The 'Essentials of Chinese Acupuncture' states that the two main functions of Xin, controlling Xue and Xue Mai, and housing Shen★, are closely related to the colour, form, motility and sense of taste of the tongue; the tongue is said to be the mirror of Xin. If Xin Qi and Xin Xue are abundant, the tongue is normal red and moist; if not, the tongue may be pale and flabby in the case of Deficient Xin Qi, or pale thin and dry in the case of Deficient Xin Xue. Stagnant Xin Xue may show as purplish colouration of the tongue; and Blazing Xin Fire may result in dry red tongue, with soreness and ulcerations. Disturbance of Shen★ by Phlegm Heat may involve a rigid tongue, that is difficult to move, leading to stuttering. Hence, disharmonies of Xin may cause disturbances of speech, such as difficult or incoherent speech, stuttering or aphasia.

Patterns of Disharmony

Patterns of Xin disharmony may be divided into two groups; those associated with underlying Yang Deficiency, and those associated with underlying Yin Deficiency:-

Yang Deficiency	Yin Deficiency
Deficient Xin Qi	Deficient Xin Xue
Deficient Xin Yang	Deficient Xin Yin
Stagnant Xin Xue	Blazing Xin Fire
Cold Phlegm Misting Xin	Phlegm Fire Agitating Xin

The foundations of Xin pathology are the Xin functions of Ruling Xue and Xue Mai, and of housing Shen*. Deficient Xue circulation and Deficient Shen* are associated with patterns of Deficient Xin Qi, Yang and Xue. Deficient Xin Yang may lead to Stagnant Xin Xue, due to Deficient Xue circulation, since Yang is needed to move Xue. Movement of Shen* may be obstructed by Phlegm, or disturbed due to Deficient Xue or Deficient Yin, and especially by Blazing Xin Fire or Phlegm Fire.

Origins
The origins of the different Xin disharmonies are illustrated in Figure 10.3.

Deficient Xin Qi

Signs
This pattern includes general signs of Deficient Qi, for example, pale face, shortness of breath on exertion, spontaneous sweating intensified by exertion, lethargy, weak pulse, and pale flabby tongue. It also includes the specific Xin sign of palpitation.

Pathology
The general signs of Deficient Qi reflect the strong relationship between Qi and Fei, as discussed on page 139. For example, since Fei Qi and Xin Qi are linked via Zong Qi, Deficient Xin Qi shows signs such as shortness of breath and palpitation, since Deficient Zong Qi will affect both respiration and heartbeat.

Also, since Xin Qi moves Xue, Deficient Xin Qi may result in weakness and irregularity of the pulse, reflecting in such pulse patterns as knotted or intermittent.

Treatment (see Deficient Xin Yang)

Common Disease Patterns (see Deficient Xin Yang)

Deficient Xin Yang

Signs
The signs of Deficient Xin Yang are as for Deficient Xin Qi, but are often more severe, since Deficient Xin Yang may be a progression of Deficient Xin Qi, and with the addition of signs of Cold; for example aversion to Cold, cold limbs, oedema, deep weak pulse, and pale moist flabby tongue.

Figure 10.3 Origins of Xin Disharmonies

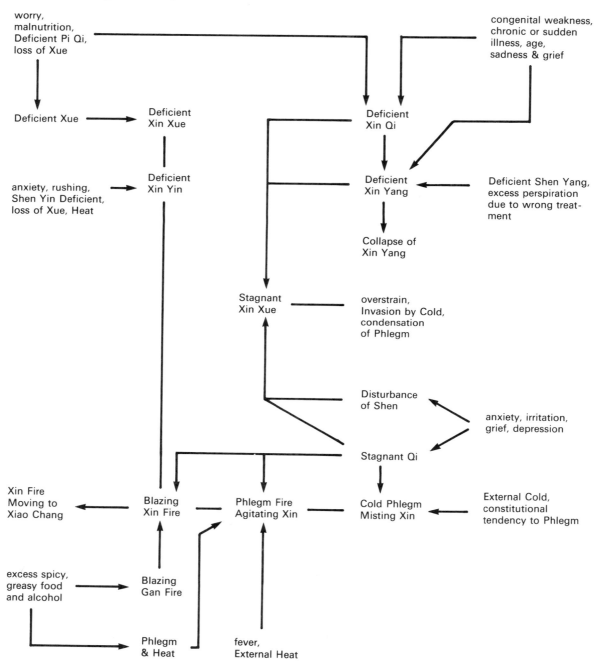

Pathology

Pathology of Deficient Xin Yang is similar to the pathology of Deficient Xin Qi, with the addition that, if Xin Yang is Deficient, circulation of Xue is impaired, leading to chilliness and cold limbs. If Deficient Xin Yang is associated with Deficient Shen Yang, Shen does not regulate Jin Ye properly, resulting in oedema.

If Deficiency of Xin Yang becomes very severe, Yang may collapse, with signs of profuse sweating, extreme cold in the limbs or entire Body, cyanosis of lips, and loss of consciousness, with minute or imperceptible pulse. Yin and Yang may separate, and the patient may die.

The Yang Qi is very weak, resulting in extreme perspiration, due to lack of control of the pores, and extreme Cold, due to lack of movement of Qi and Xue. Failure to move Xue results in cyanosis and minute pulse. Collapse of Xin Yang results in lack of nourishment of Xin, which fails to house Shen*, with loss of consciousness.

Differentiation between the patterns of Deficient Qi, Deficient Yang, Deficient Xin Qi and Deficient Xin Yang, is outlined in Table 10.1.

Table 10.1 Comparison of the Signs of Deficient Qi, Deficient Yang, Deficient Xin Qi and Deficient Xin Yang

Deficient Qi	Deficient Yang
bright pale face; spontaneous sweating; shortness of breath; lethargy; weak pulse; pale tongue	signs of Deficient Qi, but more severe; plus signs of Cold, e.g. aversion to Cold, cold limbs, deep pulse; tongue moist
Deficient Xin Qi	**Deficient Xin Yang**
signs of Deficient Qi; plus palpitations; + knotted or intermittent pulse	signs of Deficient Yang; plus palpitations; + knotted or intermittent pulse

Treatment

For chronic heart disease associated with Deficiency of Xin Qi and Xin Yang, a variety of points may be used to strengthen Xin Qi and Xin Yang and Shen Yang; using reinforcing method and moxa. Moxa is especially applicable if Xin Yang is the predominant Deficiency.

Points may be selected from such as the following:-

Jianshi, P.5, Neiguan, P.6, Tongli, HE.5, Shenmen, HE.7, Shaofu, HE.8, Xinshu, BL.15; all of which strengthen Xin and pacify Shen*. Qihai, Ren 6, may be used to strengthen Qi and Yang, and Guanyuan, Ren 4, to strengthen Shen Qi and Shen Yang. Shanzhong, Ren 17, may be added to strengthen Zong Qi, Xin Qi and Xin Yang.

Common Disease Patterns

Arryhthmia, cardiac insufficiency, coronary arterio-sclerosis, angina pectoris, general weakness, nervous disorders and shock.

Stagnant Xin Xue

Signs
The pattern of Stagnant Xin Xue shows such signs as:- stabbing pain or stuffiness in the heart region, in which pain may be referred to the left shoulder and arm, or along Xin Jing Luo; purple face and cyanosis of lips and nails, palpitations, lassitude, shortness of breath, cold extremities, and choppy, knotted or wiry pulse, and purple tongue perhaps with purple spots.

Pathology
Just as Deficient Xin Qi may progress to Deficient Xin Yang, the latter may progress to Stagnant Xin Xue; so that all these three conditions may occur together. Here we have signs of Deficient Qi:- lethargy, and shortness of breath; of Deficient Yang:- cold extremities; of Deficient Xin Qi:- palpitation and knotted pulse; and of Deficient Xin Yang:- cyanosis due to lack of Yang to move Qi and Xue. Deficiency of Xin Qi and Yang, if severe, may impair the flow of Xin Xue to the point where there is stagnation and obstruction of Xue, in the Body in general and in Xin in particular. This stagnation results in pain and stuffiness in the heart region, which may be accompanied by discomfort along the course of the Xin channel. The impaired circulation and stagnation of Xue also results in the purple face, tongue, lips and nails; and in the choppy pulse. The wiry pulse reflects not only the Stagnation of Xue, but also the pain associated with it, and is further emphasised when the condition is aggravated by Invasion of External Cold.

Pain is the sign that differentiates this pattern from the other Xin disharmonies. If Phlegm contributes to the Xue Stagnation, there may be sensation of stuffiness in the chest as well as, or instead of pain, in addition to such Phlegm signs as greasy tongue coat.

When this pattern is preceded by Deficient Xin Yang, it is an example of Deficiency complicated by Excess.

Treatment
For angina pectoris, associated with Stagnation of Xin Xue, the principle of treatment during the attack is to stimulate Xue circulation to remove stagnation, and to reduce Phlegm. Between attacks the principle of treatment is to strengthen Xin Yang and warm Shen and Pi. Reducing method is used during the attack, and between attacks reinforcing or even method is used with moxa. Points such as the following may be used during the attack:-

Ximen	P.4	Xi point of Xin Bao channel, promotes circulation in the channels and collaterals of the chest to remove stagnation and pain. Important in acute heart disease and pain, and is specific for angina pectoris. Pacifies Shen*.
Geshu	BL.17	Influential point for Xue, invigorates Xue circulation, reduces Phlegm.
Shanzhong	Ren 17	Invigorates circulation of Qi and hence of Xue to remove stagnation and Phlegm, especially in combination with Geshu.

Between attacks, points such as the following may be used:

Neiguan	P.6	Regulate Qi of Xin and Xin Bao channels, and
Jueyinshu	BL.14	reinforces Yang.
Pishu	BL.20	
Zusanli	ST.36	Warm Yang of Pi and Shen to Transform the Phlegm.
Shenshu	BL.23	
Taixi	KID.3	

Common Disease Patterns
Angina pectoris, myocardial infarction.

Deficient Xin Xue

Signs
The signs of this pattern include:- dull pale complexion, vertigo, insomnia, dream-disturbed sleep, poor memory, restless, anxiety, the state of being easily frightened, palpitations, thin pulse and pale tongue.

Pathology
The dull pale complexion, pale tongue and thin pulse are signs of Deficient Xue; since there is insufficient Xue to fill and to nourish face, pulse and tongue. Vertigo may be a sign of Deficient Yin or Deficient Xue, but when in combination with the former signs, indicates Deficient Xue. Palpitations indicate, in this case, that there is insufficient Xue to fill and to nourish Xin. Insomnia, dream-disturbed sleep, poor memory, restlessness, anxiety and the state of being easily frightened, are signs that there is insufficient Xin Xue to house Shen★ so that Shen★ is Disturbed.

Treatment
Deficient Xin Xue may occur with or without Deficient Xin Yin. If alone, moxa may be used; if with Deficient Xin Yin, moxa should be avoided. In the case of insomnia due to Deficient Xin Xue, the principle of treatment is to strengthen and regulate Xin and Pi. The following points may be used with reinforcing method:-

Anmian	N-HN-54	Specific for insomnia.
Yintang	M-HN-3	Specific for dream-disturbed sleep.
Shenmen	HE.7	Calm Xin and Shen★, invigorate circulation of Qi and Xue.
Xinshu	BL.15	
Sanyinjiao	SP.6	Strengthen Pi to produce Xue.
Pishu	BL.20	

In addition, the relatives of the patient may be asked to moxa Yintang and Yongquan KID.1, on the patient before sleep. Moxa is used here in insomnia due to Deficient Xue, but may not be appropriate for insomnia due to Deficient Yin or conditions of Excess.

129

Common Disease Patterns

Common disease patterns for this disharmony are:- insomnia, anaemia, severe malnutrition, and depressive neuroses such as postnatal depression following haemorrage during or after childbirth.

Deficient Xin Yin

Signs

There are general Yin Deficient signs such as low fever, night sweating, malar flush, hot sensation in palms and soles, dry mouth, thin rapid pulse, and dry red tongue with no coat. In addition there is the specific Xin sign of palpitation, and signs of Disturbed Shen*, such as insomnia, dream-disturbed sleep, feelings of unease and restlessness, anxiety and irritability.

Pathology

There are palpitations and signs of Disturbance of Shen*, as with Deficient Xin Xue, but, in addition, there are signs of Deficient Yin and of Heat. When this pattern is associated with Deficient Shen Yin, it is called 'Xin and Shen not Harmonised'.

A vicious circle is often set up, since living life in a perpetual stressed rush and hurry can originate and greatly aggravate Deficient Xin Yin, and on the other hand, Deficient Xin Yin can give rise to the feelings of unease, restlessness and anxiety, that originate or aggravate the tendency to rush. This disharmony is common in women manifesting a Deficient Yin type of menopausal pattern, and may be accompanied by Deficient Shen Yin and Deficient Gan Yin.

Treatment

The principle of treatment is to strengthen and nourish Xin Yin and pacify Shen*. If accompanied by Deficiency of Yin of Shen and Gan, Shen Yin must be nourished, and Hyperactive Gan Yang and Blazing Gan Fire pacified. If accompanied by Deficient Xin Xue, then Xue and Xin Xue must be nourished. Reinforcing method is used without moxa.

For example, in insomnia resulting from disharmony of Xin and Shen, the following points may be used:-

Shaofu	HE.8	Pacifies Xin Fire and calms Shen*.
Xinshu	BL.15	Pacificies Xin and Shen*.
Shenshu	BL.23	Strengthens Xin.
Yingu	KID.10	Strengthens Xin and dispels Heat.
Taixi	KID.3	Strengthens Shen Yin.
Fengchi	GB.20	May be added if Xin Fire is accompanied by Rising Fire of Gan and Dan.

Common Disease Patterns

This pattern may be involved in the following:- arrhythmia, tachycardia, hypertension, hyperthyroidism and anxiety neurosis.

Blazing Xin Fire

Signs
The signs of this pattern include:- restlessness, irritability, insomnia, feelings of heat, flushed red face, thirst, bitter taste, dark urine, pain and/or bleeding on urination, mouth and tongue ulcers, full rapid pulse, and red tongue, especially with red tip, central crack, and thin yellow coat.

Origins
This pattern may be a progression of Deficient Xin Yin, or may arise during some fevers by Invasion of Xin Bao by pathological Heat, and External Heat may contribute here. Severe emotional irritation and stagnation can result in Disturbance of Shen*, and in Stagnation of Qi, which may then give rise to Fire. In addition, excess consumption of spicy, greasy food, may result in Heat and Phlegm, with Blazing Gan Fire, which may then originate or aggravate Blazing Xin Fire.

Pathology
This is a condition of Excess Heat, with feelings of Heat, flushed, red face, dark urine, full rapid pulse, and red tongue with yellow coat. Heat gives rise to Disturbance of Shen*, with restlessness, irritability and insomnia, but these signs are more severe than in the case of Deficient Xin Yin.

Xin opens into the tongue, so that Blazing Xin Fire produces redness, soreness and ulceration of the tongue, especially of the tip, the area of the tongue that corresponds to Xin. The bitter taste results from Excess Fire affecting taste, which is partially controlled by Xin. It could be said that the face is red since Xin manifests in the complexion, but most patterns of Excess Heat also produce a red face. This redness is different from the malar flush of Deficient Yin, since it involves the whole face; just as the pulse is full, and the tongue has a yellow coat, in contrast to Deficient Xin Yin, where the pulse is thin and the tongue has no coat. These differences result from the difference between an Excess Heat and a Deficient Heat pattern.

If Xin Fire moves to Xiao Chang via their Internal-External Zang Fu relationship, the Fire in Xiao Chang may result in dark urine with pain and/or bleeding, and feelings of fullness in the lower abdomen.

Treatment
The principle of treatment is to pacify Xin Fire and calm Shen*, by using reducing method. For example, in glossitis associated with Blazing Xin Fire, such points as the following may be used:-

Shaochong	HE.9	Well point of Xin channel, pricked to bleed to reduce Xin Fire
Shenmen	HE.7	In combination with Shaochong, reduces Xin Fire and Calms Shen*.

In addition, Zhongji, Ren 3, may be used, with reducing method, to eliminate Damp Heat in the Lower Jiao, if Heat has shifted to Xiao Chang. Sanyinjiao and

Taixi may be used with even method to strengthen Yin, and to support Xin Yin in order to counteract the effects of Xin Fire.

Common Disease Patterns

This pattern may be involved in glossitis and hyperthyroidism. It also commonly occurs in combination with other patterns, for example, with Blazing Gan Fire in hypertension and hyperthyroidism, with Fire in Xiao Chang in some haematurias, with Deficient Shen Yin and Deficient Xin Yin in some forms of insomnia, and with Phlegm Fire agitating Xin in various forms of manias.

Table 10.2 Comparison of the Signs of Deficient Xue, Deficient Yin, Deficient Xin Xue, Deficient Xin Yin and Blazing Xin Fire

Deficient Xue	Signs Common to Deficient Xue and Deficient Yin	Deficient Yin
dull pale face; weak tremors in limbs; scanty menses; pale tongue & lips	emaciation; dizziness; spots in visual field; thin pulse	malar flush; warm palms and soles; night sweats; agitation; rapid pulse; red tongue
Deficient Xin Xue	Signs Common to Deficient Xin Xue and Deficient Xin Yin	Deficient Xin Yin
Deficient Xue signs; plus signs of Disturbance of Shen*; plus palpitations	signs of Disturbance of Shen*:- unease, insomnia, forgetfulness; plus palpitations	Deficient Yin signs; plus signs of Disturbance of Shen*; plus palpitations
	Blazing Xin Fire	
	signs of Excess Heat:- whole face red, full rapid pulse, red tongue with yellow coat; plus tongue ulceration, severe insomnia & agitation; ± dysuria & haematuria	

Phlegm Fire Agitating Xin

Signs

This pattern may involve signs of insanity, raving incoherent speech, violent behaviour, laughing and crying without reason, perhaps loss of consciousness, slippery rapid pulse, and red tongue with yellow greasy coat.

Pathology

This pattern of Excess has similar origins to that of Blazing Xin Fire, but with a major difference; the predominance of Phlegm, and the effects of the combination of Phlegm and Fire on consciousness and the balance of mind and emotions.

Signs such as insanity and violent behaviour result from the combination of extreme Disturbance of Shen* due to Heat, and obstruction of Shen* due to Phlegm. The Orifices of Xin are said to be obstructed, which in severe cases can lead to loss of consciousness due to obstruction of movement of Shen*.

The red tongue with yellow coat and the rapid pulse are due to Heat, and the greasy tongue coat and slippery pulse are due to Phlegm.

Treatment (See Cold Phlegm Misting Xin)

Common Disease Patterns (See Cold Phlegm Misting Xin)

Cold Phlegm Misting Xin

Signs
Muttering to oneself, aphasia, depression, introverted manner, staring at walls, lethargic stupor, rattling sound in throat, sudden loss of consciousness; slippery slow pulse; and tongue with white greasy coat.

Pathology
Like the previous category, this is an Excess pattern in which Xin is obstructed by Phlegm, but in this case the Phlegm is associated more with signs of Cold than with signs of Heat. It is a Yin rather than a Yang Excess pattern, which is reflected in the signs of mental and emotional imbalance, which are more Yin and inward and less Yang and extrovert, than in the case of Phlegm Fire agitating Xin. These signs are caused by Phlegm obstructing the movement of Shen*, which, when severe, may cause loss of consciousness. The rattling in the throat, slippery pulse, and greasy tongue coat, reflect Phlegm in the Body; and the slow pulse and white tongue coat reflect Cold.

The extreme forms of these two excess Phlegm patterns may be differentiated as follows:-

Table 10.3 Comparison of Signs of Cold Phlegm Misting Xin and Phlegm Fire Agitating Xin

	Cold Phlegm Misting Xin (Phlegm Cold)	Phlegm Fire Agitating Xin (Phlegm Fire)
Yin Yang	relatively Yin	relatively Yang
Cold Heat	Cold signs e.g. slow pulse & white tongue coat	Heat signs e.g. rapid pulse & yellow tongue coat
Mental signs	relatively introvert & depressive, e.g. staring at walls, muttering to oneself; lethargic stupor	relatively extrovert & manic, e.g. violence, shouting, laughing & crying; incessant or incoherent talking
Common Disease Patterns	windstroke sequellae; depressive psychosis; speech & mental retardation in children	severe, violent insanity; e.g. hysteria & manic psychosis

However, Table 10.3 creates an artificial distinction, since in practice the two patterns may alternate, oscillate, or transform into each other. Phlegm Fire agitating Xin may be sub-divided into Yin and Yang types, and Phlegm Misting Xin may show some Heat signs. Also, both patterns may be complicated by the involvement of Gan Wind, and in the case of Phlegm Fire agitating Xin, Blazing Gan Fire also.

133

Treatment

The principle of treatment is to clear the Orifices of Xin and Orifices of the Senses by resolving Phlegm; for Phlegm Fire agitating Xin, eliminate Heat and calm Shen⋆; and for Cold Phlegm Misting Xin, open the channels to allow the suppressed emotions to flow.

For example, in manic psychosis, points such as the following may be used:-

Hegu	LI.4	Disperse Heat from Yangming channels.
Quchi	LI.11	
Shaoshang	LU.11	Disperses Heat, clears the mind, dispels madness.
Daling	P.7	Reduce Heat in Xin Bao channel, cool Xin.
Laogong	P.8	Eliminates Phlegm and calms Shen⋆.
Jianshi	P.5	
Taichong	LIV.3	Pacify Gan Yang, Fire and Wind, cleanse the
Fengchi	GB.20	Yang which has been obscured by Phlegm, Pacify
Dazhui	Du 14	Shen⋆ and clear the Brain.
Dingshen	N-HN-32	Specific for psychosis.
Fenglong	ST.40	Strengthens Pi to resolve Phlegm, calms Shen⋆.

In depressive psychosis, points such as the following may be used:-

Renzhong	Du 26	Clears the Senses and calms Shen⋆.
Bahui	Du 20	Clears the Senses and calms Shen⋆, stabilises the ascending Yang.
Sishencong	M-HN-1	Joined to Bahui, augments its action.
Yamen	Du 15	Clears the Senses and consciousness, especially for incomplete maturation of the Brain and stiff tongue inhibiting speech.
Yiming	M-HN-13	Combines with Yamen for incomplete maturation of the Brain.
Tongli	HE.5	Regulates Xin Qi, clears Xin, pacifies Shen⋆, specific for aphasia.
Neiguan	P.6	Invigorates Wei and Xin, pacifies Shen⋆.
Fenglong	ST.40	As above.

For 'mania', manic psychosis, reducing method is used; for 'insanity', depressive psychosis, even method is used, and moxibustion may be applied if appropriate.

Common Disease Patterns

This pattern may be seen in disharmonies such as aphasia, epilepsy, speech or mental retardation in children, Windstroke sequellae, hysteria, manic and depressive psychoses.

Summary

The individual Xin disharmonies often occur together in groups and are often interwoven with the patterns of other Zang Fu. For example, Deficient Xin Qi and

Yang often occur together, sometimes with Deficient Qi and Yang of Pi and Shen, sometimes with Stagnation of Xin Xue.

Deficient Xin Xue may occur with Deficient Xin Qi, with Deficient Pi Qi and general Xue Deficiency; or with Deficient Xin Yin, perhaps accompanied with Deficient Yin of Shen and Gan. Blazing Xin Fire may occur with Deficient Yin of Shen, Gan and Xin; with Blazing Fire of Gan; and with Fire in Xiao Chang. Cold Phlegm Misting Xin and Phlegm Fire Agitating Xin may occur with Hyperactive Gan Yang, Blazing Gan Fire and Gan Wind; so that the effects of Phlegm, Wind Heat and Yang disturbance may be inextricably interwoven.

Xin patterns may be of Deficient Yin or Deficient Yang, Cold or Heat, Deficiency or Excess, or they may be Deficiency complicated by Excess, as in the case of Stagnant Xin Xue. However, in the main, the origins of Xin Disharmony are Internal rather than External.

Table 10.4 Xin Patterns of Disharmony

Pattern	Signs	Pulse	Tongue
Deficient Xin Qi	bright pale face; shortness of breath; spontaneous sweating; palpitations	weak ± knotted or intermittent	pale
Deficient Xin Yang	as Deficient Shen Qi, but more severe; plus cold limbs & aversion to Cold	weak slow ± knotted or intermittent	pale, moist
Collapse of Xin Yang	as Deficient Shen Yang, but more severe; extreme perspiration; extreme cold limbs cyanosis	minute	purple
Stagnant Xin Xue	stabbing pain in heart region; purple face, cyanosis of lips & nails; palpitations	choppy knotted ± wiry	purple ± purple spots
Deficient Xin Xue	dull pale face; unease; insomnia; palpitations	thin	pale
Deficient Xin Yin	malar flush; night sweats; agitation; insomnia; palpitations	thin rapid	red, dry; no coat
Blazing Xin Fire	whole face red; tongue ulceration; extreme agitation; ± haematuria & dysuria	full rapid	red; yellow coat
Phlegm Fire Agitating Xin	violent insanity; raving; incoherent speech; laughing & crying without reason	slippery rapid	red; greasy yellow coat
Cold Phlegm Misting Xin	muttering to oneself; depression; blank expression, aphasia; rattling sound in throat	slippery slow	greasy white coat

Xiao Chang

Functions

Xiao Chang receives the transformation products of food and drink from Wei, and has the function of 'Separating the Pure from the Impure'. The clear fraction is extracted by Xiao Chang and sent to Pi, and the turbid fraction is sent downwards to Da Chang.

Xiao Chang is involved in Jin Ye metabolism, since it sends some of the impure fluids it receives from Wei, to Shen and Pang Guang for separation and excretion, under the control of Shen Yang.

In physiology and pathology, Xiao Chang has very close links with Pi, Wei and Da Chang, and with Shen and Pang Guang. The link between the Zang system Xin and its traditionally paired Fu, Xiao Chang, is rather tenuous, and mainly manifests when Heat from Fire in Xin shifts into Xiao Chang and moves downwards, disturbing the Lower Jiao.

Patterns of Disharmony

Deficient Cold in Xiao Chang is equivalent to Deficient Pi Qi, discussed on page 87, and **Stagnant Qi of Xiao Chang** corresponds to Stagnation of Cold in Gan channel, discussed on page 119. This leaves two main disharmonies:-

Obstructed Qi of Xiao Chang
Excess Heat in Xiao Chang

Obstructed Qi of Xiao Chang

This roughly corresponds to the Western syndrome of acute intestinal obstruction, which in TCM, is associated with Stagnation of Qi and Xue, Cold or Heat, or parasites collecting in the intestines and blocking passage.

Signs include violent pain in the abdomen, no passage of gas or faeces, and perhaps vomiting of faecal material. Pulse is wiry and full and tongue has a greasy yellow coat.

The principle of treatment is to eliminate blockage and to open the intestines, using strong stimulation, i.e. reducing method. Points may be selected from the following:-

Qihai	Ren 6	Invigorates Qi circulation.
Zhongwan	Ren 12	Invigorates Pi and Wei Qi, relieves retention of food.
Shangjuxu	ST.37	Lower Uniting point for Da Chang, regulates Wei and Intestines.
Xiajuxu	ST.39	Lower Uniting point for Xiao Chang, regulates Xiao Chang.
Tianshu	ST.25	Alarm point of Da Chang, in combination with Shangjuxu and Xiajuxu for clearing obstruction from Intestines.

Excess Heat in Xiao Chang

This has already been mentioned under Blazing Xin Fire on page 131. For example, in haematuria due to downward movement of Heat from Xin to Xiao Chang, signs may include polyuria, dysuria, haematuria, irritability, feeling of fullness in lower abdomen; rapid slippery pulse; and red tongue with yellow coat. The principle of treatment would be to eliminate Heat from Xin, and from the Lower Jiao. Reducing or even method is used; points may be selected from such as:-

Tongli	HE.5	Luo point of Xin with Xiao Chang, to clear Heat from Xin.
Yinlingquan	SP.9	Eliminate Damp Heat from Lower Jiao and regulate Pang Guang.
Sanyinjiao	SP.6	
Zhongji	Ren 3	

Table 10.5 Xiao Chang Patterns of Disharmony

Pattern	Signs	Pulse	Tongue
Obstructed Qi of Xiao Chang	violent abdominal pain; no passage of gas or faeces; perhaps vomiting of faeces	wiry full	greasy yellow coat
Excess Heat in Xiao Chang	feeling of fullness in lower abdomen; polyuria, dysuria, haematuria; irritability; sore throat	rapid slippery	red; yellow coat

Chapter
11

Fei (Lungs) and Da Chang (Large Intestine)

Fei

Functions

1. Rules Qi and Governs Respiration
2. Dispersing and Descending Function
3. Moves and Adjusts the Water Channels
4. Rules the Exterior of the Body
5. Opens into the Nose; Manifests in the Body Hair

Rules Qi and Governs Respiration

Governs Respiration
Zong Qi, Qi of the Chest, gathers in the chest, forming a Sea of Qi. It is responsible for the movements of respiration and of the heartbeat, and aids Fei in the circulation of Qi, and Xin in the circulation of Xue.

Under the influence of Zong Qi, Fei governs the inhalation of the pure Qi of air, and the exhalation of the impure Qi of air. If Zong Qi and Fei functions are harmonious, respiration is smooth and regular; if Fei or Zong Qi are weak or obstructed, respiration is impaired and the Dispersing and Descending functions of Fei are affected.

Rules Qi
Fei is invloved in both the formation and the movement of Qi. As shown in Figure 3.6, on page 18, Gu Qi, derived from food and drink by the action of Pi and Wei, is sent up by Pi to Fei, where it combines with the pure Qi of air, to form Zong Qi

and Zhen Qi, under the influence of Xin and Fei. Zong Qi assists Fei in the movement of Qi around the whole Body, i.e. it assists Fei in the Dispersing and Descending functions. If Fei is weak, and the formation and movement of Qi is impaired, there may be Deficiency or Stagnation of Qi in any part of the Body.

Since Zong Qi regulates both Fei and Xin, the relationship between the Fei function of movement of Qi and the Xin function of movement of Xue is very close. In addition, there is the basic relationship in which Qi moves Xue and Xue nourishes Qi. It is in this sense that Fei is said by some texts to control Xue Mai.

Dispersing and Descending Functions

The Dispersing and Descending functions of Fei are concerned primarily with the movement of two Substances: Qi and Jin Ye. Movement of the latter is the topic of the next sub-section, here we are mainly concerned with the movement of Qi.

Dispersing Function

The Dispersing, disseminating or circulating function of Fei, is concerned with the spreading of Qi throughout the Body. Zhen Qi, formed in Fei, has two facets, Wei Qi and Ying Qi. Fei assists the dispersal of Wei Qi through the Muscles and the skin, mainly outside of the Jing Luo; and the dispersal of Ying Qi throughout the Body, mainly within the Jing Luo, including the Xue Mai.

The Dispersing action of Fei, similarly assists the spreading of Jin throughout the skin and Muscles, flowing with the Wei Qi; and the distribution of Ye to the Zang Fu, joints, Brain and Orifices, flowing with the Ying Qi.

Failure of the Dispersing function may lead to Deficiency and Stagnation of both Qi and Jin Ye throughout the System.

Descending Function

Since Fei is the topmost Zang, the natural direction of movement of its Qi is downwards. However, there is a specific relationship between Fei and Shen, described on page 70, whereby Fei sends Qi down to Shen, which receives it and holds it down. If Fei does not properly send down the Qi, or if Shen fails to hold it, Qi rebels upwards, impairing both the Dispersing function of Fei, and the proper rhythm of respiration.

Also, in the cycle of Jin Ye circulation shown in Figure 7.2 on page 69, and discussed in the next sub-section, Fei liquefies the impure fluids and sends them down to Shen for separation and excretion. Shen vaporises a part of the Jin Ye it receives and sends it back up to Fei. Failure of Fei to send down the impure Jin Ye from circulation results in oedema and may affect the Dispersing function also.

Moves and Adjusts the Water Channels

Fei receives the pure fractions of the Jin Ye from Pi as vapour, separates them, and circulates them throughout the Body. There are three main fractions: going to the skin, to the Body and to Shen, respectively. The first two, purer fractions, circulate as vapour; the lighter fraction Jin, to the skin and Muscles, and the denser fraction Ye, to the interior of the Body, as previously described. Fei liquefies that part of the circulating Jin Ye that has become impure through use, and sends it down to Shen. So the Dispersing function of Fei circulates the purer fractions of the Jin Ye as vapour, whilst the Descending function sends the impure fraction down as liquid.

If the Fei functions of Dispersing and Descending Jin Ye become weak then there may be excessive or deficient perspiration, due to impairment of the dispersing of Jin and Wei Qi to the skin; and general or local oedema, especially in the upper Body, due to the Deficiency of both the Descending and the Dispersing functions.

Rules the Exterior of the Body

Fei is the topmost Zang, 'the Lid of the Yin Organs', and is considered the 'Tender Organ', since it is the Zang in most direct contact with the external environment, and the Zang most easily invaded by External Disease Factors.

Also, Fei assists the Dispersing of Wei Qi and Jin to the Muscles, skin and surface of the Body, and is responsible not only for the moistening, nourishing and warming of the skin, but also for the regulation of perspiration and resistance of the Body to External Factors.

If Fei Qi is weak, and the Dispersing function Deficient, the protective function of Wei Qi will be reduced, and External Disease Factors are more likely to enter the Body.

Opens into the Nose; Manifests in the Body Hair

The brilliance of Fei is said to manifest in the body hair. This is an aspect of the function of Fei to rule the Exterior, since the Exterior, in this context, includes skin, body hair, sweat glands, and resistance to External Invasion. If Fei Qi is weak, and the skin and body hair are not properly moistened and nourished, the skin may be rough, dry and flaccid; the body hair poor and lustreless; and the pores may not open and close properly.

Fei opens into the nose, the pathway for respiration, via the throat, the 'Door of Fei' and the residence of the vocal cords.

If Fei Qi is weak, and there is impairment of the respiratory, Dispersing, moistening or protective functions of Fei, there may be blockage or inflammation of nose and throat, and disorders of the vocal chords.

The sign of Deficient Qi, low, weak voice, with little desire to speak, relates to both the role of Fei in ruling Qi, and to control by Fei of the vocal chords. Sudden loss of voice usually reflects invasion of Fei by External Disease Factors.

Patterns of Disharmony

Deficient Fei Qi
Deficient Fei Yin
Invasion of Fei by Wind
Retention of Phlegm in Fei

Since Fei Rules Qi, it may be associated with Qi Deficiency. Since Fei needs moisture for proper functioning, it is susceptible to External or Internal Heat or Yin Deficiency, producing Dryness. If Fei Qi is weak, failure of the Dispersing function may lead to Stagnation of Qi and Jin Ye in Fei, with accumulation of

Phlegm. Since Fei is closely linked to the Exterior, if the Dispersing function is weak, and there is inadequate circulation of protective Wei Qi, Fei may be invaded by External Pathogenic Factors.

Origins

The origins of Fei disharmonies are summarised in Figure 11.1. Fei disharmonies can be classified according to the Eight Principles' Patterns:-

Yin-Yang, Internal-External, Deficiency-Excess, and Cold-Heat.

Figure 11.1 Origins of Fei Disharmony

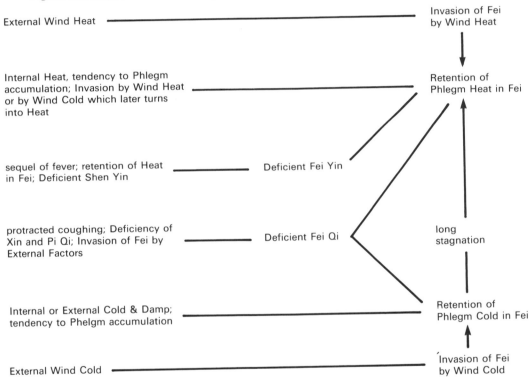

Firstly, Yin Yang; Deficient Fei Yin may be associated with Deficient Shen Yin and with Deficient Yin of other Zang Fu. The tendency to Phlegm accumulation may be associated with Deficient Shen, Pi and Fei Yang, and possibly also with Deficient Xin Yang, if Yang Deficiency is severe and general. Whereas Deficiency of Yin is associated with Heat and Dryness, Deficiency of Yang in this case is associated with failure of Pi function of proper Tranformation and Transportation of Jin Ye, and failure of Fei function of Dispersing and Descending. As a result, Damp accumulates in Fei, and may condense as Phlegm.

Deficient Qi, Yang and Yin are Internal conditions, but they may predispose to Invasion of Fei by External factors, or they may be aggravated by them. The main External factors here are Wind, Heat, Cold and Damp, which may invade Fei in various combinations.

Deficient Qi, Yang and Yin are conditions of Internal Deficiency. If these conditions lead to invasion of Fei by External Factors, and the latter accumulate in Fei; or if the Internal conditions lead to accumulation of Internal Damp and Phlegm, the Deficient conditions may turn into Excess. Excess conditions may simply be caused by invasion by, and retention of, External Factors, but usually there is a predisposing Internal Deficiency, enabling invasion by External Factors to occur.

Deficient Fei Qi

Some texts do not list the category of Deficient Fei Qi, but include it in the categories of invasion of Fei by Wind and Retention of Phlegm in Fei. There is a reciprocal relationship between Deficient Fei Qi and the Invasion and Retention patterns, since Deficient Fei Qi may predispose these patterns, which in their turn may originate or aggravate Deficient Fei Qi. In other words, the Deficiency, Invasion and Retention phenomena may all be part of the same pattern, which manifests different facets, depending on Internal and External conditions.

Signs
Signs of Deficient Fei Qi include:- weak cough, weak voice and lack of desire to talk, shortness of breath aggravated by exertion, weak respiration, asthma; copious, clear dilute sputum; fatigue, pallor, spontaneous daytime perspiration, lowered resistance to invasion by for example Wind Cold; weak pulse, and pale tongue with thin white coat.

Pathology
The signs of Deficient Fei Qi are almost identical to the signs of Deficient Qi (see page 21). This is due to the very close relationship between Fei and Qi, already discussed on page 139.

The signs of weakness are due to Deficiency, specifically of both Qi and Fei. The disharmonies of Respiration — shortness of breath, and asthma and cough — are due to the failure of the function of Fei in governing respiration, and in sending down the Qi to Shen. Hence, the breathing movements are no longer strong and even, and Qi rebels upwards, causing cough and asthma. The sputum is copious and dilute, since Deficient Fei Qi may be predominantly associated with Deficient Fei Yang, and Deficient Yang is associated with copious, clear, dilute secretions. In this case, Deficiency of Fei Qi and Yang are associated with weakness of Fei function of Dispersing and Descending of Jin Ye, with accumulation of Jin Ye and some condensation into Phlegm.

Since Fei governs vocal chords, there is weak voice and lack of desire to talk. Since Fei governs the Exterior, there may be spontaneous daytime sweats and lowered resistance to invasion, due to failure of Fei in proper Dispersing of Wei Qi to the pores and the Body surface. The patient may suffer from frequent colds, a manifestation of Deficient Fei Qi and Yang, and Deficient circulation of Wei Qi with Invasion of the Body by Wind and Cold.

Treatment
This pattern is usually found in combination with others, for example with Deficient Shen and Pi, Qi and Yang, as in the Deficient Yang form of pulmonary tuberculosis; or with Invasion of Fei by Wind and Retention of Phlegm in Fei, as in bronchitis.

Treatment will depend on which Zang Fu are involved; and whether the condition is acute or chronic, Hot or Cold, External or Internal. It will also depend on whether there is Invasion or Retention of External Factors, on whether the Deficient pattern has turned into Excess; and on the specific needs of the patient at that time. Possible points for the common cold and for bronchitis, are given on pages 145 and 147, dealing with Invasion of Fei by External Wind, and Retention of Phlegm in Fei respectively.

Common Disease Patterns
Deficient Fei Qi may be involved in:- bronchitis, asthma, pulmonary tuberculosis, emphysema, common cold and allergies.

Deficient Fei Yin

Signs
Signs of Deficient Fei Yin may include general signs of Yin Deficiency, such as:- afternoon fever, night perspiration, hot sensation in palms and soles, malar flush, emaciation; thin rapid pulse; and red tongue, perhaps with thin dry coat. In addition there may be signs of dry unproductive cough; or cough with scanty sticky sputum, which may be tinged with blood; dry itchy throat; and low hoarse voice.

Pathology
The general Yin Deficiency signs are those of Dryness and Heat, and the signs of Yin Deficiency specific to Fei manifest as Dryness and Heat in the respiratory system, for example, dry throat and dry cough. If Yin Deficiency develops into Fire in Fei, then this may damage the blood vessels and there may be haemorrhage, resulting in blood-stained sputum or in epistaxis.

Treatment
The principle of treatment is to clear Heat from Fei, and strengthen Yin of the Body and of Fei. For pulmonary tuberculosis associated with Deficiency of Yin and Hyperactivity of Fire, points such as the following may be used with even or reducing method:

Dazhui	Du 14	Disperses Heat, reduces fever.
Zhongfu	LU.1	
Kongzui	LU.6	Disperse Fire in Fei.
Feishu	BL.13	
Geshu	BL.17	Keeps Xue in Xue Mai.
Yinxi	HE.6	Eliminates Heat and reduces night sweats.
Shenmen	HE.7	Calms Xin and Shen*, to reduce irritability and insomnia.
Sanyinjiao	SP.6	Nourish Yin.
Taixi	KID.3	

Common Disease Patterns
Deficient Fei Yin may be involved in:- chronic bronchitis, bronchiectasis, chronic pharyngitis, pulmonary tuberculosis.

Dryness of Fei

Some authorities mention this minor category, often seen in some areas of China in autumn and winter when the weather is dry. This is an External pattern due to Invasion of External Dryness, which does not necessarily involve Deficiency of Yin or signs of External Heat, as in Deficient Fei Yin. The invasion is seasonal, and of short duration, with such External signs as headache and fever, and signs of Dryness in Fei, such as dry nose and throat, dry cough with no or scanty sputum, and with red-tipped tongue with thin yellow coat. In the experience of the author, a similar pattern may be produced by sleeping in a room with a dry, hot atmosphere, such as that produced by storage heaters.

Invasion of Fei by Wind

Of all the Zang, Fei is the most sensitive to Invasion by External Factors; the most important of which are Wind Cold and Wind Heat, which may transform into each other.

Signs
Signs of Wind invasion are itchy throat, cough, headache, fever and chills, sweating, aversion to wind, and superficial pulse.

If Wind is associated with Cold, chills are more prominent than fever, sweating may be less or absent; in addition to aversion to Wind there is aversion to Cold, and pulse is not only superficial but also tight. Also, there may be asthma, nasal obstruction, watery nasal discharge, cough with thin watery sputum; and tongue with thin white coat.

If Wind is associated with Heat, fever is more prominent than chills, and perspiration may be increased. There may be signs of Heat and Dryness in Fei such as red sore swollen throat; asthma; full cough with yellow sticky sputum; and dry nose, perhaps with bleeding. In addition, there may be general signs of Heat, such as: thirst, constipation, dark urine, pulse rapid as well as superficial; and red tongue with thin dry yellow coat.

Pathology
Invasion of Fei by External Wind affects the Dispersing and Descending functions of Fei, and hence the process of respiration in all areas of the respiratory system, with itchy throat and coughing. External Wind invades the superficial part of the Body, with derangement of the protective Qi, leading to opening of the pores, sweating, aversion to Wind, and superficial pulse. The headache results from invasion of the Tai Yang channels by External Wind, and the fever from the struggle between Wei Qi and External Wind. The failure of Wei Qi to warm the skin and Muscles leads to chills.

144

The association of Cold or Heat with Wind involves the additional presence of Cold or Heat signs, such as copious or scanty sputum, or slow or fast pulse. Both External Heat and External Cold may affect the Dispersing and the Descending functions of Fei, resulting in cough, asthma or nasal obstruction, which will be associated with signs of Cold and Excess fluids in the case of Wind Cold, and of Heat and Dryness in the case of Wind Heat.

Treatment

The common cold is an example of Invasion of Fei by Wind. The principle of treatment is to disperse Wind, and to disperse Cold in the case of Wind Cold, or to disperse Heat in the case of Wind Heat. Principal points such as the following may be used:-

Hegu	LI.4	Disperses Wind Cold, and especially Wind Heat; in combination with Fuliu causes sweating to relieve External signs.
Lieque	LU.7	Luo point of Fei channel strengthens Dispersing and Descending functions of Fei, disperses Wind, especially Wind Cold; especially effective in combination with Waiguan.
Waiguan	TB.5	Connecting point of San Jiao and Yang Wei channels, disperses External conditions especially Wind Cold.
Fengchi	GB.20	Intersection of Dan and Yang Wei channels, and since Yang Wei controls the external Yang, Fengchi disperses External conditions, for example of Wind Cold or Wind Heat, relieving Headache, nasal congestion etc.

Additional points for Wind Cold may be added to the principle points chosen:-

Fengfu	Du 16	Eliminate Wind and External signs, relieve
Fengmen	BL.12	headache.
Feishu	BL.13	Strengthens Dispersing and Descending functions of Fei, eliminates Wind and Exterior signs.
Fuliu	KID.7	With Hegu, causes sweating to aid relief of External conditions.

Additional points for Wind Heat may be added:-

Shaoshang	LU.11	Prick to cause bleeding, to disperse Wind Heat in the Fei channel, and ease the throat.
Dazhui	Du 14	Relieves Wind and External conditions, disperses Heat.
Quchi	LI.11	Disperses External conditions and Heat.

Further additional points may be added for specific conditions, such as headache, nasal congestion, and so on. Reducing method is used for all points. In addition, cupping may be used on points of the upper back and neck.

Common Disease Patterns
Invasion of Fei by Wind may be involved in either acute conditions, or in acute flare-ups of chronic conditions, such as:- common cold, pneumonia, bronchitis, asthma, tonsilitis.

Retention of Phlegm in Fei

'Pi forms Phlegm, Fei stores it.' There is a reciprocal relationship between accumulation of Phlegm and failure of Dispersing function of Fei; each may originate or aggravate the other.

Phlegm is a secondary disease factor, derived from Internal or External Damp. It may take time for Phlegm to condense from Damp and to accumulate. Since Phlegm has a tenacious and material aspect, it gradually takes longer to accumulate and disperse than Wind Cold or Wind Heat. It is associated with conditions of obstruction, stagnation and retention, and is a progression from Damp, just as Stagnant Xue is a progression from Stagnant Qi.

Phlegm may originate Internally, associated with chronic Deficiencies of Qi and Yang of Shen, Pi and Fei; and, especially in this case, may be slow to disperse, since these chronic Deficiencies may respond slowly to treatment. Phlegm may originate Externally, by Invasion of Fei by Wind Heat, Wind Cold or by Damp, resulting in an Excess condition. This External invasion may be predisposed by Internal Deficiency, or, External Invasion may weaken Fei Qi, which is Excess turning into Deficiency.

Signs
Retention of Phlegm in Fei includes such signs as:- coughing or asthma with copious sputum, rattle in throat, fullness of chest; perhaps loss of appetite, nausea and vomiting; slippery pulse, and tongue with thick greasy coat.

In addition, there may be signs of Heat or Cold, depending on whether the Retention of Phlegm Damp in Fei is predominantly of Phlegm Cold or Phlegm Heat.

Table 11.1 Retention of Phlegm Damp in Fei

	Phlegm Cold	Phlegm Heat
Sputum	white	yellow
Cold/Heat	signs of Cold & perhaps Internal Deficiency	signs of Heat
Pulse	slippery & slow	slippery & rapid
Tongue coat	greasy & white	greasy & yellow

Pathology
Phlegm obstructs the movement of Qi throughout the respiratory system, impairs the Dispersing and Descending functions of Fei, and leads to the above signs. Phlegm may also obstruct the chest, with coughing, fullness and discomfort; and

Wei, with digestive disturbance. The slippery pulse and greasy tongue coat reflect the accumulation of Phlegm in the Body.

Predominance of Heat or Cold leads to predominance of signs of Heat or Cold, for example feverishness with rapid pulse and yellow tongue coat, or chilliness with slow pulse and white tongue coat. In addition, there may be signs of Internal Deficiency, especially of Pi and Fei, for example, loose stools, low voice, and weak respiration.

Treatment

The principle of treatment is to strengthen the Dispersing function of Fei Qi to disperse Phlegm. In addition, it may be necessary to disperse Wind Heat, Cold or Damp; or to strengthen Deficiency, for example of Shen Yang and Pi Yang. Generally, even method or reducing method is used to disperse the Disease Factors, and reinforcing method is used to strengthen Deficiency, but the particular methods used will depend on the situation.

For bronchitis, principal points such as the following may be selected:-

Taiyuan	LU.9	Strengthen Fei and Disperse Phlegm.
Feishu	BL.13	
Fengmen	BL.12	This combination eliminates Wind and
Hegu	LI.4	disperses External conditions.
Fenglong	ST.40	Strengthens Pi and Wei to resolve Phlegm.

If Heat predominates, points such as Dazhui, Du 14, and Quchi, LI.11, may be added to disperse Heat. If Cold due to Deficiency predominates, points such as Shenshu, BL.23, and Pishu, BL.20, may be used with moxa to strengthen the Deficiency and enable Pi to transform the Phlegm.

For nausea, Zhongwan, Ren 12, and Neiguan, P.6, may be added to pacify Wei; the former to help transform Phlegm, and the latter to open the chest.

Common Disease Patterns

Retention of Phlegm in Fei may be involved in the following diseases:- chronic bronchitis, bronchial asthma, bronchiectasis.

Summary

Patterns of Fei disharmony can be summarised by looking at the common sign of **coughing**. In true TCM, there is no symptomatic treatment of coughing. Treatment depends on the nature of the Pattern of Disharmony, of which coughing is a part, and on the particular needs of the patient.

In differential diagnosis, the key questions are:-

(i) What **kind** of cough?
(ii) Accompanied by what other symptoms?

Acute cough with copious clear sputum indicates Invasion of Fei by Wind Cold; and acute cough with thick yellow sputum indicates Invasion of Fei by Wind Heat. The pulses are superficial and slow, and superficial and rapid respectively. If the pulses are deeper, and the cough full and chronic, then copious white sputum may indicate retention of Phlegm Cold in Fei; and thick yellow sputum may indicate retention of Phlegm Heat in Fei. If the cough is sporadic, with sore flanks and other signs of Gan disharmony, for example wiry pulse, it may indicate Invasion of Fei by Gan Fire. If the cough is chronic, with exhalation easier than inhalation, and with lumber soreness, it may indicate Deficiency of Shen Qi and Shen Yang, with failure of Shen to grasp Qi. If the cough is weak, with asthma, low voice and frequent colds and influenza, it may indicate Deficient Fei Qi. A dry cough with dry throat may indicate Deficient Fei Yin, if accompanied by rapid pulse, malar flush, and other Deficient Yin signs; or, if accompanied by External signs and no signs of Deficient Yin, may show Invasion of Fei by External Dryness.

Figure 11.2 summarises the different patterns of coughing, and Table 11.2 summarises the Fei Patterns of Disharmony.

Figure 11.2 The Different Disharmonies Underlying the Different Types of Coughing

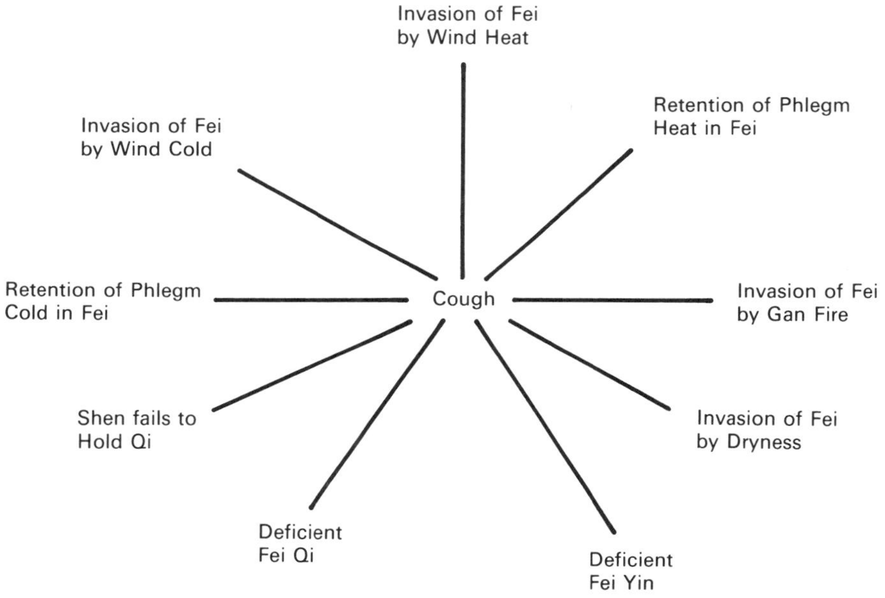

Table 11.2 Fei Patterns of Disharmony

Pattern	Signs	Pulse	Tongue
Deficient Fei Qi	weak cough; weak voice; asthma; spontaneous perspiration	weak	pale, moist; thin white coat
Deficient Fei Yin	dry, unproductive cough; malar flush; night perspiration	thin rapid	red; ± thin dry coat
Invasion of Fei by Wind Cold	itchy throat; acute cough with copious clear sputum; chills & aversion to cold	superficial tight	thin white coat
Invasion of Fei by Wind Heat	red, sore throat; thirst and acute cough; fever	superficial rapid	thin yellow coat
Retention of Phlegm Cold in Fei	cough with copious clear sputum; fullness in chest; nausea	slippery slow	thick white greasy coat
Retention of Phlegm Heat in Fei	cough with copious thick yellow sputum; fullness in chest	slippery rapid	thick yellow greasy coat

148

Da Chang

Functions

Da Chang receives the turbid fraction of the transformation products of food and fluid from Xiao Chang, moves it downward, absorbing water from it, and eliminates the remainder as faeces.

In TCM, the word Intestines may refer to both Da Chang and Xiao Chang.

Patterns of Disharmony

Although Da Chang is paired with Fei, its relationship in physiology and pathology is not so much with Fei, as with Pi, Wei and Xiao Chang. In other words, Da Chang is the final part of the digestive system, and most of the disharmonies listed under Da Chang relate to the other digestive Zang Fu. For example, **Deficient Qi of Da Chang** is often called Deficient Pi Yang, and **Cold Damp in Da Chang** is often called Invasion of Pi by Cold and Damp. The pattern called **Intestinal Abscess** approximates to the Western syndrome acute appendicitis, and the pattern of **Exhausted Fluid of Da Chang** corresponds to certain forms of constipation. The pattern of **Damp Heat Invading Da Chang** may be associated with that of Damp Heat Accumulating in Pi, with some common signs.

Intestinal Abscess

This may originate with irregular eating habits; imbalance of Cold and Heat in the abdomen, affecting Transformation and Transportation by Pi and Wei; and excess activity too soon after eating. Damp Heat accumulates in the intestines, obstructing movement of Qi and Xue, eventually forming Intestinal Abscess.

Signs are of urgent pain in the lower right abdomen, aggravated by touching, possibly fever, rapid pulse, red tongue and yellow coat. The principle of treatment is to spread the Qi in the Intestines, and to drain the accumulated Heat. Strong stimulation and continuous needle manipulation are used for 2–3 minutes, then needles are retained for 1–2 hours, with intermittent manipulation. The principal points are:-

Lanweixue	M-LE-13	Empirical point for appendicitis.
Shangjuxu	ST.37	Lower Uniting point of Da Chang.
Tianshu	ST.25	Front Mu point of Da Chang, removes obstruction and Damp Heat from Intestines, and hence relieves abdominal pain.
Zusanli	ST.36	Lower Uniting point of Wei.
Quchi	LI.11	He point of Da Chang channel disperses Heat.

Lanweixue, Shangjuxu, Tianshu and Zusanli are all on the Wei channel, which is often used for Intestinal disorders.

Dazhui, Du 14, and Hegu, LI.4 may be used in combination with Quchi, LI.11, for high fever, since these points disperse Heat. Zhongwan, Ren 12, and Neiguan, P.6 may be added for nausea and vomiting, since they harmonize Wei and suppress rebellious Wei Qi.

Damp Heat Invading Da Chang

In TCM, the Western Disease of bacterial dysentery is seen as accumulation of Damp Heat in Wei and in the Intestines from contaminated food and drink. There is diarrhoea with acute onset, and urgent need to defaecate, which continues after defaecation. Stools may have foul smell, perhaps with pus or blood, and burning sensation of anus. There may be thirst, scanty, dark urine, fever and other signs of Heat; slippery and rapid pulse; and red tongue with greasy yellow coat. In other words, there are signs of Damp and Heat affecting the Intestines, and the Body as a whole.

The principle of treatment is to disperse Damp and Heat and to harmonize Wei, Xiao Chang and Da Chang. The following principal points may be used with strong stimulation, but without retention of needles:-

Dachangshu	BL.25	Back Shu and front Mu points of Da Chang,
Tianshu	ST.25	remove obstruction and Damp Heat from Da Chang.
Shangjuxu	ST.37	Lower He point of Da Chang, combines with Tianshu to eliminate Damp Heat in Da Chang.

In addition, Zhixie, N-CA-3, may be added for diarrhoea; Neiguan, P.6, for nausea and vomiting; Quchi, LI.11, for fever; and Guanyuan, Ren 4, the Alarm point of Xiao Chang, to eliminate intestinal obstructions.

Constipation and Diarrhoea

The two signs most commonly associated with Da Chang are constipation and diarrhoea. Both of these are signs rather than diseases, and both may be associated with a wide variety of patterns. Either may be associated with Cold or with Heat, and either may be associated with Deficiency or Stagnation of Qi; however, constipation tends to be associated with Dryness, and Diarrhoea with Damp.

Depression of Gan Qi may be associated with diarrhorea directly, or via the pattern of Stagnant Food. It may also be associated with the pattern of Stagnant Qi, giving rise to constipation.

Cold may obstruct the Qi in the abdomen, resulting in constipation, or, if Cold is associated with Invasion of Damp, there may be acute onset of watery diarrhorea. Alternatively, Cold and Damp may be associated with Deficient Pi Qi and Deficient Pi Yang, and with chronic, watery, loose stools, perhaps containing undigested Food. If the chronic Internal Cold and Damp are associated with Deficient Shen Yang, there may be diarrhoea with the need to defaecate in the early morning.

150

Accumulation of Dry Heat may give rise to dry stool and constipation, but the accumulation of Damp Heat may be associated with acute onset of diarrhoea with burning anus, fever and abdominal pain.

Dryness in Da Chang may be associated with Heat or with exhaustion of Da Chang fluids, and also with Deficient Xue, resulting in constipation with dizziness and dull pale face, lips and nails. Deficient Qi is usually associated with constipation, with the patient feeling more tired after defaecation, and stools that are not dry. However, Deficient Qi of Da Chang, otherwise known as Deficient Pi Yang, may give rise to chronic diarrhoea as above.

Table 11.3 Da Chang Patterns of Disharmony

Pattern	Signs	Pulse	Tongue
Intestinal Abscess	urgent lower right abdominal pains, resisting touch; ± fever	rapid	red; yellow coat
Damp Heat Invading Da Chang	urgent defaecation; stool with pus or blood; burning anus; thirst; ± fever	slippery	red; greasy yellow coat
Exhausted Fluid of Da Chang	constipation with dry stool	thin	red, dry

Summary

The disharmonies of Da Chang are difficult to separate from those of Pi, Wei and Xiao Chang. Indeed, as seen above, the points used for Da Chang problems are those which also influence Pi, Wei and Xiao Chang; and are especially those on the Wei channel, for example, Zusanli, Shangjuxu, Lanweixue and Tianshu. Disharmonies of Shen and Gan may also influence Da Chang, especially by their affects on Pi, for example, Shen Yang Deficiency originates Pi Yang Deficiency, and Depression of Gan Qi results in Invasion of Pi.

Chapter
12

Xin Bao (Pericardium) and San Jiao (Triple Burner)

Xin Bao

Functions

The Five Zang:- Shen, Pi, Gan, Xin and Fei are the key Zang Fu in both theory and practice. Xin Bao, the sixth Zang, or Yin organ system, is of relatively little importance. Traditionally, it is the outer shield of Xin, protecting Xin from Invasion by External Pathological Factors. Xin was likened to the Emperor, who was inviolate, and Xin Bao to the Minister who guarded the Emperor from harm, and whose specific general function was guiding the people in their joys and pleasures.

The links between Xin Bao and its paired Fu, San Jiao, are particularly tenuous, and it may be that these two Zang Fu were linked more from the reason of a desire for theoretical symmetry, than from observed physiological or pathological relationships.

In clinical practice, points on the Xin Bao channel are used almost interchangeably with points from the Xin channel. Points from these two channels have very similar functions, for example to eliminate Fire or Phlegm from Xin, to move and regulate Xin Qi, to dispel fullness and pain in the chest, and to calm Xin and Shen*.

Patterns of Disharmony

The disharmonies of Xin Bao are largely connected with Warm Diseases, i.e. febrile disorders, associated with invasion of the Body by External Pathological

Heat. Just as the Pattern of Six Stages, otherwise known as the Six Divisions, was formulated for Diseases induced by Cold, the Pattern of Four Stages (Wei Qi Ying Xue), and the Pattern of San Jiao, were introduced to describe Diseases induced by Heat. Disharmony of Xin Bao is associated with the Ying or Xue stage of Wei Qi Ying Xue, and with the Upper Jiao phase of the San Jiao Pattern.

Two main Xin Bao patterns occur: one of Heat affecting Xin Bao, and the other of Phlegm obstructing Xin Bao. These patterns have comparable signs to the Xin patterns of Phlegm Fire Agitating Xin and Cold Phlegm Misting Xin, and, like them, are often interwoven with each other. However, unlike the Xin patterns, which are largely due to Internal Disease Factors, these two Xin Bao patterns are due to invasion by an External Factor, specifically Heat.

Since, it would seem, in China, treatment of the Patterns of Wei Qi Ying Xue and San Jiao is largely the province of herbal medicine rather than of acupuncture, and since the severe febrile diseases are becoming rare in the West, and even rarer in general acupuncture practice, these patterns of Invasion of Xin Bao by External Heat are of theoretical interest, but, at present, of limited practical importance in Western acupuncture.

San Jiao

San Jiao is variously known in the West as the Triple Burner, Triple Warmer, and Triple Heater. It is the sixth Fu, or Yang organ system, and is the most difficult of all the Zang Fu to understand, and the one over which there has been the most controversy, both in China and in the West. In addition, in the West, there has been an unfortunate amount of misinterpretation and misunderstanding of its role, which has further confused the issue.

All Zang Fu refer more to functions than to structures, but San Jiao is the extreme case - 'San Jiao has a name but no bodily shape.' A brief analysis of the historical development of the San Jiao concept is given in Porkert (19), and will not be considered here. The current conception of San Jiao may be considered to have the following four main facets, each of which will be discussed:-

1. San Jiao as the Three Divisions of the Body
2. San Jiao as the Fu system
3. San Jiao as the Jing Luo
4. San Jiao as the San Jiao points

San Jiao as the Three Divisions of the Body

This section may be given three subdivisions, the two less important being dealt with first.

(i)   San Jiao as part of the Six Stages
(ii)   San Jiao Classification of Warm Diseases
(iii) San Jiao as the Three Divisions

San Jiao as part of the Six Stages
In the Pattern of Six Stages, or Six Divisions, dealing with Disorders induced by
Cold, the Shao Yang stage involves Dan and San Jiao channels. However,
treatment in terms of the Six Stages is more the domain of herbal medicine than of
acupuncture, where it is of lesser clinical importance.

San Jiao classification of Warm Diseases
This is a classification of the stage or depth of invasion of Diseases Induced by
Heat, complementary to the classification of Wei Qi Ying Xue, and may be
represented as follows:-

Upper Jiao	Fei & Xin/Xin Bao
Middle Jaio	Pi & Wei
Lower Jiao	Gan & Shen

However, the treatment of severe febrile diseases is rare at present in Western
general acupuncture practice, and, like the classification of Six Stages and of Wei
Qi Ying Xue, this use of San Jiao as Three Stages or Divisions is more relevent to
herbal than to acupuncture practice.,

San Jiao as the Three Divisions
A major facet of the San Jiao concept is the idea of dividing the Body, or, more
specifically, the trunk, into three areas, the Three Burning Spaces:- the Upper,
Middle and Lower Jiao, as shown in Figure 12.1:-

Figure 12.1 The Three Divisions

Upper Jiao	Xin, Fei (head and neck)	from diaphragm upwards
Middle Jiao	Pi, Wei	between diaphragm & navel
Lower Jiao	Gan, Shen, Pang Guang Xiao Chang Da Chang	below navel

Thus, the Body is divided into three areas with respect to anatomy, physiology
and pathology.

San Jiao as the Fu System

There are three main aspects to be considered here:-

(i)   Transformation and Movement of Fluids
(ii) Transformation and Movement of Qi
(iii) Misinterpretation and Misunderstanding

154

Transformation and Movement of Fluids

The San Jiao Pathway Network

According to the 'Nei Jing', the main function of San Jiao as a Fu system, is the control and co-ordination of the formation, transformation and movements of Jin Ye. San Jiao regulates the entire cycle of Jin Ye circulation; and the inter-communication of fluids throughout the Body.

This understanding of San Jiao is very different from the concept of the division of the Body into three areas. This aspect of San Jiao suggests a network of pathways allowing the movement of Jin Ye, Qi and transformation products, throughout the Body. This pathway network may be separate from the Jing Luo of San Jiao and other Zang Fu, but integrated with them.

Closely linked to this idea of 'waterways', 'water channels' or 'water passage-ways' is, the concept of free or unobstructed movement through them. If movement is unobstructed through the San Jiao pathway network, movement of Jin Ye, Qi and transformation products proceeds smoothly. If the pathways are obstructed, then there may be accumulation of turbid fluids, with signs such as oedema or retention of urine.

The system of San Jiao pathways permeates the three Jiao, and is intimately linked with the San Jiao functions and with the internal channels and collaterals of the San Jiao, and the other Zang Fu.

Fire and Water in Jin Ye Metabolism

The fundamental division into Yin and Yang may be applied to Jin Ye metabolism. Yin corresponds to the material aspect of fluids and to their moistening, cooling and nourishing functions. Yang is the dynamic force underlying the transformation, warming and movement of Jin Ye.

The division into Water and Fire is a vital facet of the Yin Yang dichotomy. Water flows downwards, Fire blazes upwards, and a proper balance of the two represents harmony within the Body. Water corresponds to the Yin, and Fire to the Yang aspect of Jin Ye metabolism. Shen, the foundation of Yin and Yang, and of Fire and Water within the Body, has a key role in Jin Ye metabolism, and is said to Rule Water.

Jin Ye Physiology

The formation of Jin Ye is described on page 15, and the cycle of Jin Ye circulation is shown in Figure 7.2, on page 69.

The role of San Jiao in the Transformation and Transportation of Jin Ye involves:-

(i)   The concepts of Yin Yang and Fire and Water
(ii) The concepts of functional interrelationship between the Zang Fu involved in Jin Ye metabolism; principally Shen, Pi, Fei and Pang Guang, and, to a lesser extent, Wei, Xiao Chang and Da Chang
(iii) The concept of San Jiao as a network of Water Passages
(v)   The concept of San Jiao as three anatomical divisions

155

The Three Divisions and Jin Ye Metabolism

The Upper Jiao is described as a 'Mist', since it is associated with the fluid vapour that rises to Fei from Pi or Shen, and is dispersed by Fei to the skin and Muscles and to Jin Ye circulation.

The Middle Jiao is described as a 'Foam' or 'Muddy Pool', since it is associated with the process of reception and Transformation of food and drink.

The Lower Jiao is described as a 'Swamp', or a 'Drainage Ditch', since it is largely associated with the processes of excretion, carried out by Shen, Pang Guang, Xiao Chang and Da Chang.

Alternatively, the three Jiao may be regarded in terms of whether the primary concern is with the vapour phase, or with the liquid phase of fluid metabolism. The Upper Jiao is concerned with dispersing the vapour phase, and with converting impure vapour to liquid. The Middle Jiao is concerned with Transforming the solids and liquids of food and drink into a purer, lighter vapour fraction, and a less pure, denser liquid fraction. The Lower Jiao is concerned with the excretion of the impure part of the liquid phase, and with the vaporisation of the purer part of the liquid fraction.

Figure 12.2 The Three Divisions and Jin Ye Metabolism

Upper Jiao	Fei	'Mist'
Middle Jiao	Pi, Wei	'Foam' or 'Muddy Pool'
Lower Jiao	Shen, Pang Guang, Xiao Chang, Da Chang	'Swamp' or 'Drainage Ditch'

Transformation and Movement of Qi

This topic may be subdivided:-

(i)   Qi
(ii) Digestion and Excretion
(iii) San Jiao as a passage-way for Yuan Qi

Qi

San Jiao has been described as 'the beginning and end of Qi', and, as the Commander-in-Chief of the Qi of all Zang Fu, whether Ying Qi or Wei Qi, inside or outside the channels, to the right or to the left, above or below. San Jiao has been described as being responsible for communication between all parts of the Body, so that if the Qi of San Jiao is unobstructed, the Interior is harmonized and the Exterior is calmed, right and left, above and below are in communication, and the whole Body and Personality are in Harmony.

San Jiao is regarded as the source of both Ying Qi that moves through the channels, nourishing the Zang Fu, and Wei Qi, that moves outside the channels, protecting the surface of the Body from invasion by External Pathological Factors.

Digestion and Excretion

San Jiao has been described as the 'pathway for nutrition', and may be seen in terms of digestion and excretion. The Middle Jiao is responsible for the reception and 'the rotting and ripening of food and drink'. The Upper Jiao receives the purer transformation products from the Middle Jiao, and disperses them throughout the Body. The Lower Jiao receives the denser transformation products from the Middle Jiao, and mainly excretes them as waste.

San Jiao as a Pathway for Yuan Qi

According to the 'Nan Jing', the Yuan Qi from Shen, necessary to warm and activate the process of digestion, spreads from Shen to the Zang Fu via the pathway of San Jiao.

Summary

From the point of view of the San Jiao as the Three Divisions, **all** Body processes are included in the Three Divisions — not only digestion and excretion, but respiration, circulation, growth and reproduction. The Three Divisions involve the transformation and circulation not only of Qi and Jin Ye, but also of Xue, Jing and Shen. However, from the point of view of the function of San Jiao as the Fu system, the emphasis is on digestion and excretion, and the metabolism of Qi and Jin Ye. Indeed, the main function of San Jiao is the regulation of Jin Ye metabolism, and the concern with Qi and digestion and excretion is of secondary importance.

Misinterpretation and Misunderstanding

There are two main headings:-

(i)   San Jiao as a Heating System
(ii) San Jiao and the Endocrine System

San Jiao as a Heating System

In the main interpretation of San Jiao as regulating Jin Ye metabolism, there is indeed a Fire, as well as a Water, aspect. In the secondary interpretation of San Jiao as 'the avenue for food and drink and the beginning and end of Qi', warmth is both required by the digestive processes, and is produced by them. However, the Western view of San Jiao primarily as a 'Heating System' or 'Thermostat of the Body' is foreign to TCM.

San Jiao and the Endocrine System

Similarly, Western attempts to identify San Jiao with the endocrine system of Western medicine, or with specific endocrine glands, such as the thyroid, are highly inadvisable, and only lead to intellectual confusion. Firstly, TCM does not perceive an endocrine system, and, secondly, at this stage of Western understanding of TCM, attempts to equate the functional systems of TCM with the solid organs of Western medicine, only lead to gross misunderstanding and clinical inefficiency. Only when there is a deep and thorough understanding of Chinese medicine in the West can a synthesis of Western and Chinese medicine begin. That time is not yet with us.

San Jiao as the Jing Luo

Distribution
The distribution of the main superficial San Jiao channel is well-known, and only its internal pathway, and its connections with certain other systems are mentioned below. The superficial channel goes from Tianliao, TB.15, via Bingfeng, SI.12, and Dazhui, Du 14, to Jianjing, GB.21. From Jianjing, the channel goes internally to the chest, to join with Xin Bao, and connect with Shanzhong, Ren 17. It descends through the diaphragm to the abdomen, linking with the Upper, Middle and Lower Jiao in turn.

A branch of the San Jiao channel connects with Weiyang, BL.53, the lower Uniting point of San Jiao, and then follows the course of Pang Guang channel, to unite with Pang Guang.

Signs
Signs associated with the superficial pathway of the San Jiao channel include:-swelling, soreness or pain in hand, arm, shoulder, throat, cheek and jaw; pain or inflammation in eyes or ears, and deafness.

Signs associated with the internal pathway of the San Jiao channel, or with the San Jiao as a Fu system, include abdominal distension, especially hardness or fullness of the lower abdomen, urination with frequency or pain, enuresis, oedema and retention of urine.

The signs of disharmony of the San Jiao channel and of the San Jiao organ system are therefore very different; signs of the channel are mainly pain or inflammation in the upper Body, along the course of the superficial channel; and signs of San Jiao organ system are largely in the lower Body, and concerned with faulty Jin Ye metabolism.

The San Jiao Points

The San Jiao points have remarkably little association with the functions of San Jiao as an organ system. The main functions of the San Jiao points are concerned with:-

(i)   Relieving pain and inflammation along the course of the superficial channel
(ii) Dispersing External Disease Factors
(iii) Invigorating Qi circulation in the Jing Luo, to remove obstruction

Relieving the Superficial Channel
Each San Jiao point has a local effect on the area surrounding it, for example Yangchi, TB.4, is used for pain in the wrist, and Tianliao, TB.15, is used for pain in the shoulder. Also, each San Jiao point may have effect at areas on the channel, at a distance from the point, for example, Zhongzhu, TB.3, may be used for deafness, and Tianjing, TB.10, may be used for pain in the shoulder and neck.

Dispersing External Disease Factors
Various San Jiao points have the function of dispersing invading External Factors, especially Wind and Heat. For example, Waiguan, TB.5, and Sizhukong, TB.23,

158

disperse Wind and Heat. The action of these points is associated with the San Jiao function of 'harmonizing the interior and calming the exterior', and with the San Jiao as the source of Wei Qi, the defensive energy of the Body.

Invigorating Qi Circulation

Several San Jiao points are concerned with regulating or invigorating the circulation of Qi in the channels and collaterals, and hence with removing obstruction and stagnation of Qi. For example, Sanyangluo, TB.8, 'clears the channels and Sensory Orifices', and Waiguan, TB.5, removes obstruction from the Yang Wei Mai.

This aspect of San Jiao point use is associated with the concept of San Jiao as a system of passageways, which must remain unobstructed to allow the free movement of Qi, Jin Ye and transformation products. It highlights the link between San Jiao disharmonies and obstruction and stagnation.

Treatment of San Jiao Disharmonies

Points on the San Jiao channel are rarely used for San Jiao organ disharmonies. San Jiao points may be used for disorders of some of the less emphasised aspects of San Jiao functions, for example, Zhigou, TB.6, opens the Intestines, relating to the digestion and excretion aspects of San Jiao, but disharmonies of the main San Jiao function of Jin Ye metabolism are not treated by San Jiao points.

For example, in retention of urine, Zhongji, Ren 3, the Mu point of Pang Guang, may be used in combination with Sanyinjiao, SP.6, to regulate the function of Pang Guang. Weiyang, BL.53, may be added, since it is the Lower Uniting point of San Jiao, able to regulate the transformation of fluids in the Lower Jiao, and promote circulation in the Water Passages.

In oedema, obstruction of the Water Passages may be predominantly in the Upper Jiao, due to Fei disharmony; in the Middle Jiao, due to Pi disharmony; or in the Lower Jiao, due to disharmony of Shen. Treatment would depend on which Jiao and also which Zang Fu were the predominant disharmonies. For example, if Fei Qi were Deficient, Shanzhong, Ren 17, and Feishu, BL.13, could be used to strengthen it. If Pi Qi were the predominant Deficiency, Zhongwan, Ren 12, and Pishu, BL.20, could be used. If Shen Yang were the predominant Deficiency, Guanyuan, Ren 4, could be used. In each case, points would be used with both reinforcing method and moxa.

Summary

The two main conceptions of San Jiao, are of San Jiao as the Three Divisions of the Body, and of San Jiao as the Fu system. These two conceptions are not mutually exclusive, but complementary. For example, the main function of the San Jiao organ system is the regulation of Jin Ye metabolism. San Jiao as an organ system provides a system of Water Passageways which may permeate the Upper, Middle and Lower Jiao, and connect those Zang Fu involved in the cycle of Jin Ye circulation. In addition, some texts associate San Jiao as the Fu system with digestion and excretion; with the formation, transformation and circulation of Qi, and with Wei Qi and the protection of the Body from External invasion. However, the main function of San Jiao as a Fu system is with the formation, transformation, circulation and excretion of Jin Ye.

The superficial San Jiao channel has little relation to the pathology of San Jiao as a Fu system, and the points on the San Jiao channel are rarely used for San Jiao organ system disharmonies. The points used for disharmony of San Jiao as a Fu system depend on the particular Zang Fu involved, but are generally points of Jing Luo other than the San Jiao Jing Luo.

Chapter
13

Review of the Five Zang

The Twelve Zang Fu form the core of TCM, and the Five Zang are the most important of the Twelve Zang Fu. The Five Zang are:- Shen, Pi, Gan, Xin and Fei.

   If the nature and functions of each Zang are understood, then it is possible to predict which Patterns of Disharmony it will have, since the Patterns of Disharmony simply originate from failure of the functions. For example, the main function of Gan is ensuring Free-flowing of Qi. Failure of the Free-flowing of Qi results in uneven movement of Qi with obstruction, stagnation and blockage. It is

Table 13.1 Functions of the Five Zang

Shen
Stores Jing:-
  Rules reproduction & growth
  Rules Bones
Foundation of Yin Yang
Rules Water
Rules Reception of Qi
Opens into Ears; Manifests in Hair

Pi
Rules Transformation & Transportation
Rules Muscles & Limbs
Governs Xue
Holds up Organs
Opens into Mouth; Manifests in Lips

Gan
Rules Free-flowing of Qi
Stores Xue
Rules Tendons
Opens into Eyes; Manifests in Nails

Xin
Rules Xue & Xue Mai
Stores Shen*
Opens into Tongue; Manifests in Face

Fei
Rules Qi & Governs Respiration
Governs Dispersing & Descending
Regulates Water Channels
Rules Exterior of Body
Opens into Nose; Manifests in Body Hair

not surprising, therefore, that the main Pattern of Disharmony of Gan is Depression of Gan Qi.

This chapter reviews the Five Zang by observing how each Pattern of Disharmony originates from failure of a particular Zang function.

Functions

Table 13.1 lists the functions of the Five Zang, and Table 13.2 reduces this list to the main functions.

Table 13.2 Main Functions of the Five Zang

Zang	Main Function
Shen	Stores Jing
	Foundation of Yin & Yang
Pi	Rules Transportation & Transformation
Gan	Rules Free-flowing of Qi
	Stores Xue
Xin	Stores Shen★
	Rules Xue & Xue Mai
Fei	Rules Qi & Respiration
	Governs Dispersing & Descending

Interrelationships of the Main Zang Functions

Shen

Shen stores Jing and is the source of the prenatal energies within the Body. Jing governs the growth, development and senescence of all other Zang Fu, and is responsible for the transmission of the characteristics and heredity. In addition, Jing is associated with the Marrow, Bones and Brain, and is involved in the cycles of development of the Body as a whole.

Shen is the Foundation of Yin Yang, and the source of Yin Yang for each of the other Zang.

Pi

Shen Yang is the source of Pi Yang. Shen Ying and Shen Yang activate the Transportation and Transformation function of Pi, and are thus necessary for the formation of Qi, Xue and Jin Ye. However, since there is a replenishable postnatal aspect to Jing, and since Shen★ is the manifestation of Qi and Jing, Pi is also important in the maintenance of Jing and Shen★. Therefore Pi is the Foundation of Postnatal Qi, and involved in the formation and maintenance of all the Five Substances. Since Pi is responsible for the formation of Qi, Xue and Jin Ye, it rules the Flesh and the Muscles, and hence the limbs, since without the warming, nourishing and lubricating action of these three Substances, Flesh and Muscles cannot function correctly.

Gan

Gan rules Free-flowing of Qi, and hence the even movement of Qi and Xue through the Jing Luo, Zang Fu and Tissues. It also governs the regular and

162

adequate storage and release of Xue. Hence the Tendons and Muscles rely on Gan for a regular, even supply of nourishment and moisture. In this area, the functions of Pi and Gan are closely linked.

Xin

Xin stores Shen*, which is responsible for vitalizing all the systems of the Body, and contributes the unique quality of consciousness. Xin also governs Xue and Xue Mai, and is responsible for the heartbeat, the pulse and the movement of Xue through Xue Mai.

Fei

Fei is responsibile for the movement of respiration, and for the intake of the pure Qi of air from the external environment. Fei governs the Dispersing of Qi and Jin Ye around the Body, and the Descent of Qi from Fei to Shen, which is linked to the function of Shen in holding down the Qi. Fei liquefies the impure fraction of Jin Ye and sends it down to Shen; Shen vaporises the fluid and sends it up to Fei. Thus, there is a very close relationship between Fei and Shen; especially since Fei relies on Shen as the source of both Fei Yin and Fei Yang.

Fei is also closely linked to Pi, since Zhen Qi, which circulates in the Body as Yin Qi and Wei Qi, needs both Gu Qi from Pi and the Qi of air from Fei for its formation. Also, Fei is associated with the Exterior of the Body and the skin.

Obviously, although useful in giving a clear overview, this account of the main functions of the Five Zang is grossly oversimplified.

For example, each of the Five Zang is involved in the formation and transformation of Qi, Xue and Jin Ye, as shown in Table 13.3.

Origins of Patterns of Disharmony

The Patterns of Disharmony of each of the Five Zang arise from failure of a specific function or functions. If we are familiar with the nature and functions of a Zang, we can predict its Patterns of Disharmony.

Shen

The most important disharmonies of Shen are associated with Deficiency of Jing, with disorders of Bones, Brain, growth, development, reproduction and premature senility; and with relative Deficiency of Shen Yin or of Shen Yang. Deficient Shen Yin or Deficient Shen Yang may affect the other Zang, which depend on Shen for both an adequate source of Yin and Yang, and for their relative balance of Yin and Yang.

Also, if Shen Qi and Yang are weak, and Shen fails to receive Qi sent down by Fei, then there may be difficulty in breathing. Shen rules Jin Ye metabolism, and Shen Qi or Shen Yang Deficiency may manifest as Shen Qi not Firm, with leakage of sperm or urine. Alternatively, Shen Yang Deficiency may result in accumulation of fluids, and oedema, the pattern of Water Overflowing.

Pi

If Pi lacks the Qi and Yang to activate Transportation and Transformation, there may be Deficiency of Qi and Xue, and also accumulation of Jin Ye with possible

Table 13.3 The Five Zang and the Formation of Qi, Xue and Jin Ye

Zang	Qi	Xue	Substance Jin Ye
Shen	source of Prenatal Qi, activates formation of Postnatal Qi, Receives Qi from Fei	some Xue forms from Bone Marrow, activates formation of Xue	activates formation vaporisation and transformation of Jin Ye
Pi	source of Gu Qi from food & drink	source of Xue from food & drink, holds Xue in Xue Mai	source of Jin Ye from food & drink
Gan	Governs Free-flowing of Qi	ensures Free-flowing of Xue, Stores & releases Xue	ensures Free-flowing of Jin Ye
Xin	Shen★ is ultimate manifestation of Qi & Jing	Rules movement of Xue in Xue Mai	involved in inter-relationship of Xue, Yin & Jin Ye
Fei	Rules respiration & intake of pure Qi of air, Rules Dispersing & Descending of Qi	Fei & Xin are involved in formation of Xue in chest	Rules Dispersing & Descending of Jin Ye

formation of Phlegm. Also, Deficient Pi Yang may lead to inability of Pi to Hold Xue in Xue Mai, and to Hold Up the Organs. Hence, Pi depends on Shen for a proper balance of Yang.

Since Pi tends to Deficient Yang, it is susceptible to Invasion by External Cold and Damp, which in turn will further depress Transportation and Transformation. However, under certain conditions, there may be Accumulation of Damp Heat in Pi.

Gan

If the Free-flowing function of Gan becomes defective, there may be Stagnation or unevenness of movement of Qi and Xue, i.e. Depression of Gan Qi, associated with disturbance of flow of bile, digestion, emotions and menstrual cycle, and also local pain and discomfort along the course of the Jing Luo. Gan is closely linked with Pi, and if Pi is relatively Deficient, Gan may more readily invade and upset Transportation and Transformation, causing various signs of impaired digestion.

Stagnation of Qi may give rise to Heat, either Blazing Gan Fire or Damp Heat in Gan and Dan, and this may damage Gan Yin. Hence, Gan needs an adequate supply of Yin, and is easily affected by Deficient Shen Yin. Hyperactive Gan Yang may be associated with Deficient Gan Yin, and Hyperactive Gan Yang and Blazing Gan Fire may be associated with Stirring of Gan Wind. Failure of the Gan function of Storage of Xue may be associated with Deficient Gan Xue, which may also give rise to Stirring of Gan Wind.

Alternatively, Stagnation of Qi in Gan Jing Luo may be associated with accumulation of Cold and Damp.

Xin

Shen★ is subject to two main disharmonies: Deficiency and Disturbance. If Xin Qi and Yang are Deficient, there may be signs of Deficient Shen★. If Xin Xue and

Xin Yin are Deficient, there may be signs of Disturbance of Shen⋆. Also, since Xin is responsible for movement of Xue in Xue Mai, Deficiency of Qi and Yang of Xin may lead to Stagnation and Deficient movement of Xue, and specifically to Stagnant Xin Xue.

Also, since Shen⋆ must be able to move freely, if the Orifices of Xin are obstructed by Phlegm, movement of Shen⋆ will become obstructed or irregular, resulting in fluctuations of mania and depression, or loss of consciousness, as in Phlegm Fire Agitating Xin or Cold Phlegm Misting Xin.

Xin is liable to both Deficient Yin and Deficient Yang, and is therefore affected by both Deficient Shen Yin and Deficient Shen Yang. Deficient Shen Yang may be linked with Deficient Pi Yang, and hence with formation of Phlegm. This gives a combination of Deficient Shen Yang, Deficient Pi Yang and Deficient Xin Yang. Alternatively, Deficient Shen Yin may be associated with Deficient Gan Yin and with Blazing Gan Fire, and these three patterns may then originate Deficient Xin Yin and Blazing Xin Fire.

Fei

Impairment of the Fei function of Respiration may lead to Deficiency of Qi and to Deficient Fei Qi. Alternatively, Deficiency of Pi Qi and Pi Yang may lead to Deficient Qi, which then affects Fei. If Fei Qi is Deficient, then Fei cannot send Qi down to Shen, and if Shen Qi is Deficient, Shen cannot receive Qi properly, and there may be difficulty in breathing.

Deficient Fei Qi may be associated with failure of function of Fei to Disperse Qi around the Body. This may be associated with insufficient supply of Wei to the skin, and of Ying to the Muscles, so that External Disease Factors may more

Table 13.4 Patterns of Disharmony of the Five Zang

Shen	Pi
Deficient Shen Jing	Deficient Pi Qi
Deficient Shen Yang	Deficient Pi Yang
Shen Qi not Firm	Inability of Pi to Govern Xue
Shen Fails to Receive Qi	Sinking of Pi Qi
Water Overflowing	Invasion of Pi by Cold & Damp
Deficient Shen Yin	Damp Heat Accumulates in Pi

	Gan	
	Depression of Gan Qi	
	Deficient Gan Xue	
	Hyperactive Gan Yang	
	Blazing Gan Fire	
	Stirring of Gan Wind	
	Damp Heat in Gan & Dan	
	Stagnation of Cold in Gan Jing Luo	

Xin	Fei
Deficient Xin Qi	Deficient Fei Qi
Deficient Xin Yang	Deficient Fei Yin
Collapse of Xin Yang	Invasion of Fei by Wind
Stagnant Xin Xue	Retention of Phlegm in Fei
Deficient Xin Yin	
Blazing Xin Fire	
Phlegm Fire Agitating Xin	
Cold Phlegm Misting Xin	

readily invade the Body. Hence, Fei is the Tender Organ, the Zang most susceptible to External Invasion.

Invasion of Fei by External Wind is often associated with Deficient Fei Qi, and impairment of the Dispersing function of Fei. Poor Dispersing function may lead to failure to disperse the invading Factor, so that it is retained in Fei; and to accumulation of Phlegm in Fei. These Disease Factors then further impair the Dispersing function.

Fei is dependent on Shen Yang to energize its Dispersing and Descending functions. If Shen Yang and Fei Yang are Deficient, then Fei may be unable to send impure fluid down to Shen properly, or disperse Jin Ye around the Body. Since Deficient Shen Yang is associated with inability of Shen to vaporise the fluids and send them up to Fei, a combination of Deficiency of Shen Yang and Fei Yang results in breakdown of Jin Ye metabolism, and oedema.

Fei, like Xin, tends to both Deficient Yin and Deficient Yang. Deficiency of Shen Yin and Fei Yin may be associated with Heat and Dryness in Fei, and perhaps with Blazing Fire in Fei, with symptoms of dry cough and haemoptysis.

Interrelationships

Chapter
14

Zang Fu Interrelationships

The main emphasis of this book is to see the Zang Fu in terms of inter-relationships. The foundation of all interrelationship in traditional Chinese medicine is the division into Yin and Yang, and the continual process of change and transformation consequent upon it. The main components of the changing patterns of health and disease are the Substances, Jing Luo, Zang Fu and Tissues; and the Disease Factors with which these interact.

Each Zang Fu is a system of functional interrelationships, and the twelve Zang Fu together are responsible for the formation and transformation of the Substances, and their transportation inside and outside of the Jing Luo system to the Tissues and all other parts of the Body. In addition, the Zang Fu are responsible for the interaction between the individual and the environment. This involves not only the intake of nourishment and the expulsion of waste, and the balance of Wei Qi and External Disease Factors at the surface of the Body, but also the interplay between the environmental stimuli and the behaviour of the individual.

Yin Yang

The Yin Yang interaction is the primary basis of all Zang Fu inter- relationships. In disharmony, the two basic patterns are the relative Deficiency of Yin, and the relative Deficiency of Yang. Since Shen is the foundation of Yin and Yang in the Body, Deficiency of Yin or Yang of any other Zang Fu tends to originate with, or be associated with, Deficient Shen Yin or Deficient Shen Yang.

Deficient Shen Yin　　Deficient Shen Yang
Deficient Gan Yin　　Deficient Pi Yang
Deficient Xin Yin　　Deficient Xin Yang
Deficient Fei Yin
Deficient Wei Yin

Although, theoretically, every Zang Fu might have Yin Deficiency, those Zang Fu which, because of their nature, have an especial tendency towards it are Shen, Gan, Xin, Fei and Wei. It is therefore these Zang Fu which have Yin Deficiency as one of their listed patterns of disharmony.

Similarly, every Zang Fu might have Yang Deficiency, but in practice, because of their natures, only Shen, Pi and Xin have Yang Deficiency as one of their listed disharmonies.

Substances

The formation, transformation and transportation of Substances within the Body depend on the harmonious functional interrelationships of the Zang Fu. The nature, metabolism and pathology of the substances have been discussed in Chapter 3, and some of the Zang Fu interrelationships involved have been investigated in Chapter 12 on San Jiao.

In this context, the substances can be divided into two groups:-

Qi, Xue and Jin Ye
Jing and Shen

Qi, Xue and Jin Ye

Under the transforming action of Pi, the food and drink received by Wei is converted into two fractions, pure and impure. The pure fraction includes Gu Qi and fluid vapour, which rise upward, under the influence of Pi and Shen Yang, to the chest. With the involvement of Xin and Fei, and the pure Qi of air, the Gu Qi is converted into Xue, Zong Qi and Zhen Qi. Zong Qi accumulates as the Qi of the Chest, and Zhen Qi manifests as Wei Qi and Ying Qi, which circulate around the Body. The fluid vapour is dispersed, as Jin and Ye, by the action of Fei, both through the skin and Muscles, and throughout the Body. When the fluid vapour becomes impure, it is liquefied by Fei and sent down to Shen, where the purer part of it is vaporised and sent back up to Fei, and the less pure part sent to Pang Guang for processing and elimination as urine. The impure fraction produced by Pi moves down to Xiao Chang and Da Chang. The purer fractions are re-absorbed, and the impure solids expelled as faeces. Part of these impure fluids are sent to Pang Guang. The transformations that occur in Xiao Chang, Da Chang and Pang Guang, and the transportation between these sytems, are motivated by Shen Yang.

Fei governs the movement of Qi around the Body, and Xin governs the movement of Xue. The movement of Jin Ye involves Shen, Fei and Pi. All movement depends on Yang, and therefore on a sufficiency of Shen Yang. It is the function of Gan to ensure that this movement is smooth and even, and unobstructed.

Jing and Shen★
Whereas a number of Zang Fu are involved in the metabolism and movement of Qi, Xue and Jin Ye; Jing and Shen★ each relate primarily to only one organ system. Also, both Jing and Shen★ have a prenatal component, and are hence more precious and less replaceable than the other Substances. Although Jing and Shen★ are active throughout the Body, Jing is stored in Shen, and relates specifically to Shen physiology and pathology, and Shen★ resides in Xin, to which it has a special relationship.

Pathology of the Substances

The pathology of the Substances will be considered in terms of each of the Zang systems.

Shen
Shen tends not only to patterns of Deficient Yang and Deficient Yin, but also to Deficient Jing. In addition, since Shen is involved in holding the Qi sent downwards by Fei, Shen disharmonies may involve asthma or shortness of breath; and since Shen is involved in Jin Ye physiology, Shen disharmonies may involve oedema or urinary problems.

Pi
Deficiency of Pi Qi or Pi Yang may result in poor Transformation and Transportation, and hence inadequate supply of Qi and Xue, and accumulation and stagnation of turbid Jin Ye with possible condensation of Phlegm. Also, Deficiency of Pi Qi and Pi Yang may be linked with the Inability of Pi to Govern Xue, associated with haemorrhage, especially in the digestive system and lower Body.

Gan
Depression of Gan Qi may lead to Stagnation of both Qi and Xue, and Deficiency of Gan Yin may be associated with Hyperactive Gan Yang. Both Depression of Gan Qi and Deficiency of Gan Yin may develop into Blazing Gan Fire, which, if then associated with Phlegm and Rising Gan Wind, may obstruct the Orifices of Xin, with Disturbance of Shen★. If Gan loses its ability to store and regulate Xue, or if Xue becomes heated with Blazing Gan Fire, then Xue may leak from Xue Mai, and haemorrhage may occur.

Xin
Xin is involved in the formation of Qi and Xue in the Upper Jiao, but its main functions are moving Xue through Xue Mai and storing Shen★. If there is insufficient Xin Qi and Xin Yang to move Xue properly, there may be local Deficiency or Stagnation of Xue, with coldness, cyanosis or pain. If there is insufficient Xin Yin and Xin Xue to provide residence for Shen★, Shen may become disturbed, especially if there is accompanying Fire and Phlegm in Xin.

Fei
Fei is involved, along with Xin, in the formation of Qi and Xue in the chest, especially since it is responsible for respiration. However, its main functions are

the Dispersing and Descending of Qi and Jin Ye throughout the system. Fei Deficiency and Qi Deficiency are closely interwoven; failure of the Descending function may be associated with asthma and shortness of breath, failure of the Dispersing function may involve lowered resistance to invasion of the Body by External Disease Factors. In terms of Jin Ye physiology, failure of the Dispersing and Descending function may lead to oedema, and to retention and stagnation of fluid throughout the system.

Although impairment of the Dispersing and Descending functions are largely associated with insufficient Fei Yang to move the Qi and Jin Ye, they may also be associated with Deficient Fei Yin and the accumulation of Heat in Fei.

Jing Luo

The Substances, which are formed and transformed by the Zang Fu, are transported by their action to all parts of the Body. This transmission of the Substances is via three main systems:-

Jing Luo
Xue Mai
Outside Jing Luo and Xue Mai

These three systems are closely interwoven in physiology and pathology. The Jing Luo sytem is the primary concern here. Each Zang Fu has its own associated Jing Luo system:- the main channel with its superficial and deep pathways, and the Tendino-muscular, Divergent and Luo systems. The Jing Luo system of a particular Zang Fu connects the organ system to its paired Zang or Fu, to its related Tissues, Orifices and areas of the Body, and to the other Zang Fu systems.

The Jing Luo systems of all the Zang Fu together form a network through which all systems and all parts of the Body are in communication, both with each other, and with the external environment. It is via the movement of Substances through the Jing Luo system, that the physiological and pathological interrelationships of the Zang Fu are manifested.

Tissues

This heading includes three main groups:-

Tissues
Orifices/Senses
Curious Organs

Tissues
The Traditional relationships between Zang and Tissues are summarized in Table 14.1.

Table 14.1 Zang-Tissue Relationships

Zang	Rules	Manifests in
Shen	Bones	head hair
Pi	Muscles	lips
Gan	Tendons	nails
Xin	Xue Mai	face
Fei	skin	body hair

Bones and Head Hair

Marrow, Brain and Bones were discussed in relation to Jing and Shen in Chapters 3 and 7, and are considered below under the heading of Curious Organs.

Teeth

Bones, and teeth, the 'excess of the Bones', are ruled by Shen. Hence, Deficient Shen Jing may manifest in premature looseness, decay and loss of teeth; and Deficient Shen Yin may give the teeth the appearance of dry bone. However, dryness of the teeth associated with dryness, redness and swelling of the gums, may be a sign of Heat in Wei, since Wei Jing Luo is distributed to the gums; or it may be a sign of Deficient Shen Yin with Fire Blazing upwards.

Head Hair

The hair of the body is said to be ruled by Fei, and the hair of the head is said to be ruled by Shen.

Various factors combine to ensure a healthy head of hair, but two of the most important are a sufficient supply of Jing and of Xue. Deficient Jing and Deficient Xue may be associated with dull, dry hair, or with premature greying and hair loss. Abnormal hair loss, for example, may be associated with a variety of factors, including severe shock, chronic stress, malnutrition, and drug and radiotherapy. In treatment, it may be necessary, not only to strengthen Shen and Pi in order to strengthen Jing and Xue; but also to pacify Xin and Gan, to relieve tension and anxiety. The patient should be advised to avoid and reduce stress wherever possible, to reduce workload, especially of study; to get as much rest and relaxation as possible; and to take care with nutrition, perhaps taking a complete vitamin B complex to strengthen the nervous system, and iron supplement to strengthen Xue.

It is clear from this that Shen is not necessarily the only or the most important factor affecting the health of head hair; a variety of different factors may be involved, depending on the situation.

Muscles and Lips

The main area of confusion here is between the Muscles (Flesh) ruled by Pi, and the Tendons ruled by Gan. This is due to the fact that the Chinese terms, translated as Muscles and Tendons, do not correspond exactly with the Western concepts of the same name. Either Chinese term may refer to muscles, ligaments and tendons, but the use of the term Muscles implies involvement of Pi, and the use of the term Tendons implies involvement of Gan.

Pi rules the Muscles, the Flesh and the four limbs, since Pi is responsible for the formation of the Qi and Xue that nourish and moisten the Muscles. However, the

Xue available to the Muscles is also dependent on the ability of Gan to Store Xue, so that either Pi or Gan imbalance may result in poor supply of Xue to the Muscles. This situation is further complicated by the fact that imbalance of Gan and of Pi commonly occur together. For example, Depression of Gan Qi may depress the transforming and transporting functions of Pi, resulting in the aggravation of the Deficiency of Qi and Xue.

The lips are discussed along with the mouth in the section on Orifices.

Tendons and Nails

Gan is sometimes associated with the contractile aspect of muscles, ligaments and tendons, whilst Pi is sometimes associated with their bulk and strength. Thus Gan imbalance is more associated with spasm, contraction and spastic paralysis of the muscles and tendons, as in Windstroke patterns, for example CVA sequellae; whilst Pi imbalance is more associated with weakness, wasting and atrophy of the muscles and tendons, as in Wei patterns, for example myasthenia. However, according to Dr Su Xin Ming (25), there is no clear distinction between Muscles and Tendons. In Wei patterns, for example, polio, it would not be enough to treat Pi alone; points of both Pi and Gan and Dan should be used. For example, Yanglingquan, GB.34, might be used for slack muscles, due to the close relationship between Muscles and Tendons.

Nails

An adequate supply of Gan Xue ensures that the nails are pink and moist. If Gan Xue is Deficient, the nails may become thin, brittle, ridged, and pale, perhaps with white spots. Inability of Xin to move Xue to the extremities, and impairment of formation of Xue by Pi, may also affect the health of the nails.

Xue Mai and Face

Xue and Xue Mai were discussed in relation to Substances in Chapter 3, and in relation to Xin in Chapter 10. They are also briefly considered in the section on Curious Organs below. Xue is affected by disharmonies of all of the Five Zang, as shown in Table 15.3, on page 189; and Xue Mai may be affected by disharmonies of both Xin and Fei, since the movement of Xue in Xue Mai is so closely linked to the movement of Qi.

Face

The face or complexion is ruled by Xin, as mentioned on page 124. However, many other disharmonies besides those of Xin register in the face. Deficient Xue, linked with Deficiencies of Gan or Pi, may show a dull pale face; and Deficient Qi and Yang may give a bright pale face. The whole face may become red in conditions of Excess Heat or Blazing Fire; or there may be malar flush in conditions of Deficient Heat or Deficient Yin. Damp Heat in Pi or in Gan and Dan may result in a yellow, orange or greenish complexion; and Stagnation of Xue may be associated with hues of blue or purple.

Skin and Body Hair

The exterior of the body, the skin and the body hair, is said to be ruled by Fei. However, many factors, External, Internal and Miscellaneous, affect the health of the skin. The skin and the surface of the body, including the superficial Jing Luo, may be invaded by Wind, Cold, Damp, Dryness, Heat and Summer Heat, in various combinations. Internal disharmony also affects the skin. For example, Phlegm may obstruct Jing Luo, forming subcutaneous lumps which raise the surface of the skin. Swollen, puffy skin may be a sign of oedema, associated with defective Jin Ye metabolism, linked with disharmony of any combination of Shen, Fei, Pi, Wei, Xiao Chang, Da Chang, Pang Guang and San Jiao. Alternatively, dry and withered skin may represent Deficient Jin Ye and/or Xue; and fluid-filled eruptions may be a sign of Damp. Pallid skin that is loose and flaccid to the touch may be associated with Deficient Pi Qi, and with age. Skin colour may be associated with various disharmonies, as mentioned in the section on the face above. Heat may be associated with redness of the skin, as in long exposure to wind and sun, and with red eruptions or rashes. The latter are seen in TCM as Heat in Xue, and may derive from many factors: inherited predisposition, side-effects of drugs, excess 'warming' food or herbs producing Heat in the Body, exposure to External Wind and Summer Heat, emotional and mental irritation, etc.

Greasy skin and body hair may be linked with excess consumption of rich, greasy food, or with impairment of function of Zang Fu associated with digestion; Pi, Wei, Gan, Dan, Xiao Chang, and Da Chang. Greasy skin may be linked with Heat in Xue, and is often accompanied by red, pustular eruptions, associated with Damp and Heat.

In summary, Fei disharmony is only one of many Disease Factors affecting the skin, and the origins of disharmony in any patient with a skin problem must be fully understood before treatment. For example, in one patient, the following factors were combined together. There was an inherited tendency to itchy, red skin rashes, to emotional tension, and to premenstrual tension. The skin condition was worse before a period, and was aggravated by emotional tension, various cosmetics, alcohol, and by sugary, rich and greasy food. Treatment aimed at removing Heat from Xue; pacifying Gan and Xin, and strengthening Yin. The patient was asked to moderate her consumption of alcohol, avoid sweets and rich, greasy, spicy food, avoid conflict situations and to try to reduce stress; and to experiment carefully to determine which cosmetics and shampoos were safe for her.

Body Hair

Just as Shen manifests in the hair of the head, Fei manifests in the hair of the body. However, as described in the previous section on skin, Fei is not the only factor affecting body hair.

Orifices/Senses

There is considerable overlap of concepts: between Tissues and Orifices, for example, lips and mouth; and between Orifices and Senses, for example, ears as Orifices and ears as Senses.

Obviously, the healthy functioning of the Sense Organs and Orifices depends on **all** the Zang Fu working together in harmony. However, TCM proposes specific relationships between particular Zang Fu and particular Sense Organs or Orifices. These are summarized in Table 14.2, and will be considered below under the headings of the five Zang.

Table 14.2 Zang-Orifice Relationships

Zang	Orifice (Sense)
Shen	ears
Pi	mouth
Gan	eyes
Xin	tongue
Fei	nose

Shen and Ears

The upper Orifices or Sense Organs ruled by Shen are the Ears, and the lower Orifices ruled by Shen are the urethra and anus. However, according to Porkert (19), the ears are governed by both Shen and Xin, and since all Jing Luo are said to connect to the ears, various Zang Fu disharmonies may affect the ears and the sense of hearing. In pathology, Fire in Gan and Dan may generate Phlegm, and ascend to the head to disrupt the Senses. The channels of Dan and San Jiao have links with the ears, and are often used in the treatment of ear problems. Indeed, the following may be used as the main points for tinnitus:- Yifeng, TB.17, Zhongzhu, TB.3, Ermen, TB.21, and Fengchi, GB.20; and are exclusively from Dan and San Jiao channels.

Pi and Mouth

Pi opens into the mouth and manifests in the lips, so that Pi can distinguish the Five Flavours, and so that the lips are red and moist. Insensitivity to taste is generally associated with Pi, and not with the disharmonies of Xin affecting the tongue. Xin controls that aspect of the tongue concerned with speech.

However, pale lips do not necessarily indicate a chronic disharmony of Pi, they may also indicate a sudden, severe haemorrage, Deficiency of Xin Xue, or inability of Gan to store Xue properly. Also, lips that are dry and cracked may indicate not only Fire in Wei, but also febrile diseases in general. Bluish or purple lips may indicate both Deficient Xin Yang and Stagnant Xin Xue.

Gan and Eyes

All the Zang Fu contribute to the brightness of the eyes, and Shen Jing nourishes the eyes as well as the ears, but traditionally, the specific relationship is with Gan. If the eyes are bright and vital, Shen* and Jing are healthy; if the eyes are dull and lifeless, it may indicate general Deficiency of Qi and Xue, or Deficiency of Shen* and Jing. Redness of the eyes is associated with Heat, whether from External Invasion, or from Internal disharmony. Redness with exudation may indicate accumulation of Damp Heat. Exudation without redness, or muddiness of the whites of the eyes, may indicate Damp and Deficient Pi Qi. Puffiness or bagginess under the eyes may indicate Deficient Shen Qi; and so on. However, treatment of eye diseases will depend on their nature and origin, and the points used will also reflect those channels which have links with the eyes, for example, Pang Guang, Dan and Wei especially. For example, conjunctivitis is attributed in TCM to Wind and Heat, and treatment is directed to dispersing these, so that the main points may include:- Fengchi, GB.20, Hegu, LI.4, and Jingming, BL.1. Glaucoma is attributed to Deficient Shen Yin, which allows Fire and Wind in Gan and Dan to ascend. Treatment must therefore include nourishment of Yin, with such points as Taixi, KID.3, and Sanyinjiao, SP.6.

Xin and Tongue

Xin opens into the tongue, which may reflect Xin disharmony, but also, of course, reflects the disharmony of all the Zang, and hence is used as a major diagnostic procedure. For example, pale tongue does not necessarily indicate Deficient Xin Xue, it may also indicate general Qi, Yang or Xue Deficiency; and a purple tongue is not necessarily indicative of Stagnant Xin Xue, it might indicate Stagnation due to Cold, Depression of Gan Qi, or injury of Xue and Jin Ye by Heat. However, soreness and ulceration of the tongue are often associated with Blazing Xin Fire, and speech defects or disturbances may be associated with Phlegm Fire or Phlegm Cold in Xin, obstructing or disturbing Shen*. The treatment for slurred speech, for example, includes points from Xin and Xin Bao channels.

Fei and Nose, Throat and Voice

Fei opens into the nose; also the throat is the 'door' of Fei and the residence of the vocal cords. Although disharmonies of Zang other than Fei may affect the nose, since the nose is the interface between Fei and the external environment, the nose is often involved when Fei is invaded by External Factors.

Nasal disorders may be treated with local points, for example Bitong, M-HN-14, Yintang, M-HN-3, and Yingxiang, LI.20. Hegu, LI.4, may also be used, since it is a distant point on the same channel as Yingxiang, and especially since it disperses External Wind conditions. Thus, the main points used in treatment of acute rhinitis and chronic sinusitis do not include points from Fei channel, but points such as Lieque, LU.7, may be used in a supplementary capacity if Heat is accumulated in Fei.

Sore throat may be associated with various patterns, and Fei will only be treated if Fei disharmony is involved, for example, in acute tonsilitis, where Shaoshang, LU.11, is bled to disperse Heat in Fei. A weak voice with little desire to speak may be part of a Fei Qi Deficiency pattern, but is not a common presenting sign. Weakness of **voice** due to Deficient Fei Qi, is a separate phenomenon from disturbance of **speech** due to disharmony of Xin and Shen*.

Curious Organs

The Six Curious Organs are:- Bones, Marrow, Brain, Uterus, Xue Mai and Dan. They are said to resemble the Fu in form, because they are hollow, and the Zang in function, because they store and do not excrete. These tissues, in their aspect as the Curious Organs, have relatively little theoretical or practical importance, and are generally treated via other systems.

Marrow, Bones and Brain

The Yin aspect of Jing gives rise to Marrow, which may either form the Brain, the Sea of Marrow, or Bone Marrow, which may contribute to the formation of Xue. Since they are formed from Jing, and are maintained by it, all are governed by Shen, all may be involved in the pattern of Deficient Shen Jing, and all may be treated using points which strengthen Shen function.

In TCM, Xin is the seat of consciousness, since it is the residence of Shen*.

However, the Brain, and hence Shen, have a small part to play in behaviour, since the Brain is responsible for fluidity of movement, and of the senses of hearing and vision. If Marrow is Deficient, and Brain is not nourished, or if the Orifices of the Senses are obstructed, there is poor vision and hearing, dizziness and perhaps lack of consciousness. This contrasts with the disturbance of Shen* caused by obstruction of the Orifices of Xin, which is accompanied by insanity and disorders of speech. However, in certain conditions, for example mental diseases, obstruction of both Xin and Senses may occur together.

Uterus

The Uterus is the organ central to the two processes of menstruation and gestation, which are chiefly dependent on the systems of Ren Mai, Chong Mai, Shen, Pi and Gan (see page 205). Disorders of the uterus, that is of menstruation or gestation, are mainly treated using points on one or more of these five channels.

Xue Mai

There is no clear distinction between Xue Mai and Jing Luo. Both systems carry both Qi and Xue. It may be that the Xue Mai contain relatively more Xue, and Jing Luo, other than Xue Mai, contain relatively more Qi, but, in any case, although the Chinese texts devote many pages to the details of distribution of the Jing Luo, they do not detail the distribution of Xue Mai separately. Also, the points, the basic units of acupuncture treatment, are upon the superficial Jing Luo, not upon Xue Mai as a separate system.

Xin rules the movement of Xue through Xue Mai. Pi holds Xue within Xue Mai, Gan is responsible for the unobstructed even flow of of Xue within Xue Mai, and for maintaining the correct volume of Xue in circulation. In addition, Zong Qi assists Xin in its function; Shen Yang is the foundation for the Yang of the other Zang Fu, and hence for the movement of Qi and Xue; and Shen Yin is the foundation for Yin of the other Zang Fu, and hence cools Xue, to prevent it becoming hot, and leaving Xue Mai.

Dan

The functions of Dan as a Curious Organ are the same as its functions as a Fu system, which have already been discussed. It is listed as a Curious Organ, since, unlike other Fu, it stores a pure fluid, bile.

Zang Fu

This chapter has briefly discussed Zang Fu interrelationships in terms of Yin Yang, Substances, Jing Luo, and Tissues. Chapter 13 briefly considered the interrelationships of the Five Zang with each other in health and disease. The relationship between the five Zang and the Six Fu is that the six Fu are basically concerned with the digestive process, and the passing of relatively impure digestive products from one hollow organ system to another, until the least pure fractions are voided to the exterior. The five Zang are intimately associated with the six Fu in the function of digestion, but are also concerned with the storage and distribution of the pure Substances Qi, Xue, Jin Ye, Jing and Shen*.

Zang Fu Pairs

Traditionally, each of the Zang is paired with a Fu system:- Shen with Pang Guang, Pi with Wei, Gan with Dan, Xin with Xiao Chang, Fei with Da Chang, and Xin Bao with San Jiao. As mentioned on page 64, some of these pairings reflect clinical observation, for example the very close association between the Zang and Fu systems in the first three pairs; but the latter three pairs seem to have been created more to fit the theory than to fit the fact. The physical and pathological relationships between Xin and Xiao Chang, Fei and Da Chang, and Xin Bao and San Jiao, are minimal and of no great clinical importance.

A more realistic grouping of the Zang Fu could be expressed:-

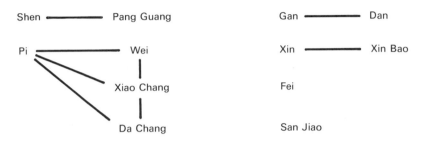

Fei, and the Xin - Xin Bao system, do not have the close relationship with a Fu system possessed by Shen, Pi and Gan; and San Jiao is more an expression of the function and relationships of other Zang Fu than a Fu system in its own right

Zang Fu and the Origins of Disease

The Zang Fu will now be considered in terms of the origins of disease. Generally, unless the External Disease Factors are extreme, and themselves weaken the Body, External Disease Factors only invade subsequent to previous weakening by other Factors. These may include trauma, previous illness, emotional disturbance and congenital weakness; or there may be a combination of a number of these Factors. In other words, if Zang Fu are strong and in harmony, the Body is healthy; and if Zang Fu are weak or in disharmony, the Body may manifest signs of disease, and be more susceptible to invasion by External Disease Factors. Thus, health and disease may be defined in terms of the harmony or disharmony of the Zang Fu and their associated Jing Luo.

The three categories of Disease Factors — External, Internal and Neither External nor Internal — have been listed in Chapter 4; and for each of the five Zang, the origins of their Patterns of Disharmony have been discussed, with outline diagrams relating Disease Factors to Patterns of Disharmony, and the different Patterns of Disharmony to each other. Later, in Chapter 16, the interrelationships of Zang Fu and Disease Factors will be looked at in more detail, in terms of the origins of specific Common Disease Patterns.

The concern here is with three patterns which may arise from the action of Disease Factors in the Body, and then, in their turn, precipitate further disharmony. These three patterns are Stagnation, Phlegm and Internal Wind.

179

Stagnation

Generally, in TCM, Stagnation implies stagnation of movement, specifically the movement of Substances, and especially the movement of Qi, Xue, and Jin Ye. The patterns of Stagnant Qi and Stagnant Xue have been mentioned in Chapter 3 on the Substances, and Stagnation of Jin Ye on page 84.

Slowing or impairment of the flow of circulating Substances may be associated with obstruction and blockage, and with the accumulation and stagnation of these Substances. This may result in local Excess, pain and swelling. Stagnation may be the result of External Cold and Damp which slow and impede the movement of Qi, but it may also facilitate the invasion of these External Factors into the Body, just as it may be associated with accumulation of Internal Cold and Damp. Indeed, Stagnation and External or Internal Cold and Damp are so closely interwoven that it is better to view them all as parts of one pattern.

Stagnation of Qi, Damp or Phlegm may eventually give rise to Heat, and to patterns of Blazing Fire, Damp Heat and Phlegm Fire respectively. This

Figure 14.1 The Main Zang Fu and Disease Factors Associated with Stagnation

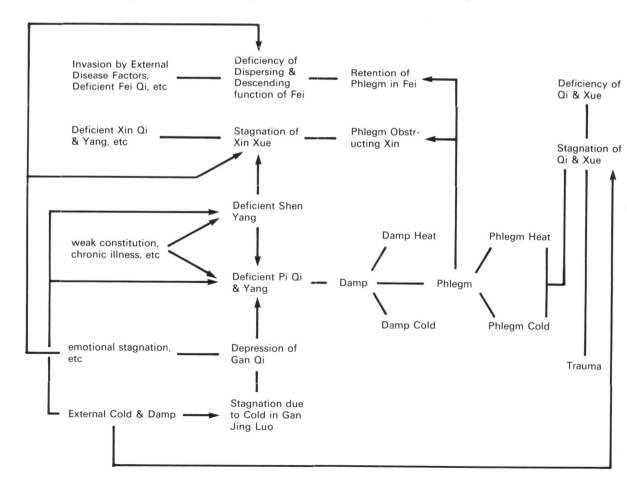

transformation may be aggravated by the presence of Internal or External Heat; and there is a close relationship between Stagnation, External Heat, Damp and Phlegm. The Zang Fu show Patterns of Disharmony of Stagnation and Cold, for example Stagnation of Cold in Gan Jing Luo; and of Stagnation and Heat, for example Damp Heat in Pang Guang. Some Zang Fu have patterns of Stagnation of both Heat and Cold types, for example, Fei may retain both Phlegm Heat and Phlegm Cold, and Xin may have patterns of Cold Phlegm Misting Xin or Phlegm Fire Agitating Xin.

Some of the main origins of Stagnation are outlined in Figure 14.1. Stagnation may arise from Deficiency of Qi and Xue, or it may give rise to these patterns. Trauma may result in the retardation in the flow of Qi and Xue in an area of the Body, and this weakened area may then be invaded by External Disease Factors, or form a focus for problems such as Bi patterns (arthritis), at a later date, for example, when age and overwork have resulted in general weakness in Qi and Xue circulation. Deficiency of the Yang of the Body, the dynamic force that assists movement, will result in retarded circulation of Qi and Xue and hence, perhaps, in Stagnation. This may be manifest as Deficient Shen Yang, and if this then results in Deficient Pi Yang, there will be impairment of Transformation and Transportation, with Deficiency of Qi and Xue, and possibly also accumulation and Stagnation of Jin Ye, forming patterns of Damp and Phlegm. Pi is said to form Phlegm, and Fei to store it. Hence, if the Dispersing and Descending functions of Fei are reduced, and weakness of Pi leads to production of Phlegm, this may accumulate in Fei, and lead to further impairment of Dispersing and Descending. Alternatively, Phlegm may obstruct the Orifices of Xin, or Deficient Qi and Yang of Xin may result in Stagnation of Xin Xue. Since Xin governs movement of Xue, and Fei governs movement of Qi, factors that affect Zong Qi, for example chest injury or emotional depression, may give rise to Stagnation of Qi and Xue.

The Zang perhaps most strongly associated with stagnation is Gan. Depression of Gan Qi associated with the impairment of the Gan function of maintaining free, smooth, even and unobstructed flow of Qi, may be associated with Stagnation of both Qi and Xue. Just as emotional Stagnation may originate Depression of Gan Qi, or may arise from it, so Stagnation of Qi and Xue may be the origin or the effect of Depression of Gan Qi.

External Cold and Damp may, over a long period, depress Shen and Pi Yang, and thus depress both movement of Substances in general, and the metabolism of Jin Ye in particular. Damp and Phlegm may then accumulate, with further Stagnation in the system, in Xin or Fei, or in Jing Luo generally. Wind, Cold and Damp may invade specific areas with local retardation and Stagnation of Qi and Xue, and this occurs especially where other factors, for example trauma, have already weakened circulation.

In addition, patterns of Stagnant Xue may arise in certain febrile conditions, for example, the Stagnant Xue which may occur in puerperal fever, and which is termed Heat Invading the Uterus.

Phlegm

Phlegm has been discussed in some detail under Pi (page 84) and under Gan (page 116). Basically Phlegm arises from Deficiency of the Transformation and

Transportation functions of Pi, resulting in accumulation and Stagnation of turbid Jin Ye, which eventually condenses as Phlegm.

Phlegm may occur as sputum in the respiratory system, or as 'Insubstantial Phlegm' obstructing Orifices of Xin or Senses. It may obstruct the flow of Qi in Jing Luo, causing numbness or paralysis, or Phlegm may accumulate, forming subcutaneous lumps, or enlargement of glands.

Phlegm may be associated with External Wind Cold as in facial paralysis; with Internal Cold and Damp, as in Deficient Shen and Pi Yang; with Heat and Fire, as in Phlegm Fire Agitating Xin; or with Fire and Wind, as in Blazing Gan Fire and Stirring of Gan Wind. Itself a product of Stagnation, Phlegm leads to further Stagnation in the Body.

Internal Wind
Internal Wind has been discussed in Chapter 9 on Gan, and its relationship with Phlegm on page 116. Stagnation, Phlegm and Internal Wind may be closely interrelated, and two Zang in particular are involved, Gan and Pi. Deficiency of Pi with the resulting accumulation of Damp and Phlegm, may result in Stagnation of the movement of Qi. Depression of Gan Qi may invade Pi, and aggravate Deficiency of Pi Qi, and also directly result in Stagnation of Qi and Xue. The Stagnant Qi may eventually give rise to Heat, for example to Blazing Gan Fire, leading to the Stirring of Gan Wind. The Hyperactive Gan Yang, Blazing Gan Fire and Gan Wind, may rise up the Body in combination with Phlegm, obstructing the Orifices of the Senses and the channels of the head, with signs of insanity or loss of consciousness.

Summary

Interrelationship forms a basic theme throughout this book. This chapter examined the interrelationships of the Zang Fu with each other and with the Disease Factors, in terms of Yin Yang, Substances, Jing Luo and Tissues.

The next chapter considers Zang Fu interrelationships in terms of emotional disharmony.

Chapter
15

Emotions

The Emotions and Behaviour

The degree of harmony between an individual and the environment is reflected in the behaviour of the individual. Harmonious behaviour depends on three closely interwoven factors:- physical health, a balanced flow of the emotions, and proper development of the intellectual faculties.

In this chapter, the emotions are artificially separated from the other components of behaviour for convenience of study. The word emotions, as used here, refers to the fluid movement of feelings, as experienced by the subject, and as manifested by their behaviour; as in anger, fear, jealousy, grief, and so on.

However, the emotions are not necessarily pathological factors; the changing flow of the emotions is part of healthy behaviour, varying with environmental pressure, inherited tendency, age, stage of development, and other factors. Emotions are only associated with disharmony when their flow becomes obstructed or irregular, when they become deficient or excessive, or when one or more become abnormally predominant over the others. Emotional imbalance may then give rise to Zang Fu disharmony. Alternatively, disorders of the Zang Fu may result in Emotional disturbance, and often a vicious circle is set up:-

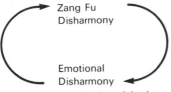

For example, an imbalance of Gan may give rise to anger and depression, which, in turn, aggravate the imbalance of Gan.

This relationship between Zang Fu disharmony and emotional imbalance, will manifest in the behaviour of the individual, perhaps creating environmental disturbance which then aggravates the Internal disharmony of the individual, or, elaborating the vicious circle:-

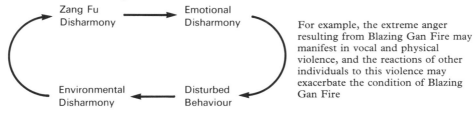

For example, the extreme anger resulting from Blazing Gan Fire may manifest in vocal and physical violence, and the reactions of other individuals to this violence may exacerbate the condition of Blazing Gan Fire

Within the Body, emotional disharmony is associated with disturbance of the function of Zang Fu in the formation and transformation of Substances, and with disturbance or obstruction of their movement, via Jing Luo, between the different organ systems and Tissues. The normal emotions and the emotional disharmonies associated with each of the five Zang are considered below.

Classifications of the Emotions

Table 15.1 The Seven Emotions
Qi Qing

Chinese word	English words
Xi	joy, happiness, gaiety, excitement, pleasure
Nu	anger, irritation
Si	meditation, contemplation, pensiveness
You	anxiety, sorrow
Kong	fear, extreme anxiety
Jing	sudden intense fear, fright
Bei	grief, affliction

Table 15.2 The Five Feelings
Wu Zhi

Chinese word	English words	Zang associated
Xi	joy, etc.	Xin
Nu	anger	Gan
Si	meditation, etc.	Pi
You	anxiety	Fei
Kong	fear	Shen

Sometimes, You, anxiety, sorrow is omitted from the Seven Emotions, and Si is split into two:- Si, worry, and Yu, anxiety. Hence, worry is often associated with Pi and anxiety with Fei. Furthermore, Bei, affliction, grief, is often included along with You, sorrow, anxiety in Fei. Also, there is not complete agreement as to which emotion is associated with which Zang Fu; for example, some consider worry damages Fei, others consider worry injures Pi. Some group sadness with Deficiency of Xin and lack of joy with Deficiency of Shen★, and suggest it injures Xin, others group sadness with grief and sorrow, and suggest it damages Fei.

All this ambiguity merely reflects the fluidity of the emotions which are constantly rising and falling, and merging and transforming into each other. There are many shades of emotion and it is not possible to give them all precise and rigid names. Some, for example anger and fear, are basic, and come into nearly every list. But the Five Feelings or Seven Emotions do not even give enough primary emotions, let alone the full range of shades and nuances. For example, where are pride, greed, jealousy, cruelty, hate, vengefulness, envy and so on? There are other systems which are more flexible and extensive (2 and 26), but no system of classification of the emotions can be wholly satisfactory.

The Five Feelings and the Five Zang

Fear and Shen

The emotion of fear is strongly linked to self-preservation, the will or desire to live. Following the stimulus, there are sensations of fear, fright and terror, and there may be temporary loss of control of defaecation and urination. There may be immobility, the paralysis of fear, or the attempt to escape from the danger — flight, or to combat it — fight. Each of these three possibilities may be appropriate in particular circumstances. Paralysis may be associated with weakness of Dan — the paralysis of indecision; and fight may be associated with the linkage of the emotions of fear and anger, and of Shen with Gan.

Extreme fear has obvious survival value, it is sudden and temporary. However, the continual stress of modern living may result, in some individuals, in a state of fearful anxiety which is less extreme but chronic. This may be linked with feelings of panic in joint disharmony of Shen and Xin, with worry in disharmony of Shen and Pi, and with anxiety in disharmony of Shen and Fei.

Also, fear may be of a wide range of phenomena:- of being in enclosed spaces, of being alone, of not being loved, of sex, of the unknown, and so on. Indeed, in the opinion of the author, the limited language of the Five Feelings and Seven Emotions is wholly inadequate to deal with the subtleties and complexities of emotional disharmony.

Shen is associated with the emotions of fear and fright. If they are extreme, then Shen Qi may descend, and the individual may temporarily lose control of urination and defaecation, since Shen governs the Lower Orifices, the urethra and anus. Extreme or chronic fear may injure Shen. However, Dr J. H. Shen is of the opinion that grief affects Shen (23), and that when grief is locked inside and not outwardly manifested, Xin Qi is weakened and Shen Qi is damaged.

Anger and Gan

Anger, associated with Gan, is linked with a violent bursting out of emotion. The accompanying sound is shouting, and the mode of action is wrenching and pulling. Bursts of anger may be accompanied by bright red face and trembling of the muscles. However, although anger may be closely associated with fear, there may be a distinction between 'shivering with fear', and 'shaking with rage'.

Failure of the Free-flowing function of Gan, Depression of Gan Qi, may be associated with frustration and depression, and periodic outbursts of anger. This may arise if there has been much frustration and obstruction of the feelings and actions of the individual, so that the chronic frustration may result in alternate anger and depression.

Deficient Gan Yin and Hyperactive Gan Yang are more associated with feelings of edginess, irritability, and moderate anger; and these Gan disharmonies may arise from chronic irritation and annoyance, especially if the individual is already feeling hypersensitive. Blazing Gan Fire is linked with severe and violent outburst of rage.

Anger may also arise from being frightened, threatened, insulted or injured. The allied emotions of hatred, resentment, intolerance and so on are beyond the scope of this discussion.

Joy and Xin

Happiness, associated with Xin, can be that wonderful feeling of lightness and release, following successful resolution of a long-term frustration and difficulty. In this sense, joy is the child of anger, as in the Mother-Son relationship of Five Phase Theory. But, joy may also be associated with excitement, laughing, talking, and general social hyperactivity. Also, joy may be associated with pleasure, languor, sensual enjoyment. There are many levels and facets of this emotion.

Excess joy is said to injure Xin, since it scatters the Xin Qi, so that Shen* becomes confused and disordered. According to Dr Shen, excess joy over- expands Xin, just as shock and fright may over-contract it.

Deficient Shen* may be associated with dullness, apathy, lack of vitality and lack of joie de vivre. However, it may be difficult to separate lack of joy from depression due to Depression of Gan Qi, and from sadness, sorrow and melancholy associated with disharmony of Fei.

The two Zang most concerned with maintaining a balance of the emotions, and the two most susceptible to emotional disturbance are Gan and Xin. Gan is responsible for maintaining a smooth and even flow of the emotions, and if Gan is disharmonious and there is irregularity and obstruction of this flow, the emotions may become extreme, fluctuating and inappropriate. Xin is responsible for housing Shen*, and if Shen* becomes obstructed or disturbed, there may be extremes of depression or mania. The most extreme disturbances of emotion and of behaviour arise from disharmonies of Gan or of Xin.

Pensiveness and Pi

Si, the emotion associated with Pi, is variously described as pensiveness, cogitation, contemplation and meditation. It is said that excess thinking, excess study, obsessive thinking and worry injure Pi, and may depress the functions of Transformation and Transportation involved in digestion.

Some Western texts have associated Si with sympathy, the emotion of caring, compassion and enfolding, but in the experience of the author, Chinese sources refer more to pensiveness than to sympathy.

Grief and Fei

Grief, associated with Fei, is the pain of loss, the pain of letting go. Associated with it are the related emotions of sorrow, melancholy and loneliness. In TCM, anxiety is also linked with Fei.

Whether sadness is included in this list, or interpreted as a lack of joy and associated with Deficiency of Shen*, is perhaps unimportant, since all these related emotions will tend to stagnate the Zong Qi in the chest, and hence weaken the function of both Fei and Xin. This may result in weakness and stagnation of Qi and Xue throughout the body.

According to Dr Shen, worry injures Fei, since unhappiness and worry weaken the breathing.

186

The Five Feelings and the Five Phases

Students of the major Western colleges are familiar with basic Five Phase Theory, which is ably discussed elsewhere (12), and will not be debated here.

Figure 15.1 The Five Feelings and the Five Phases

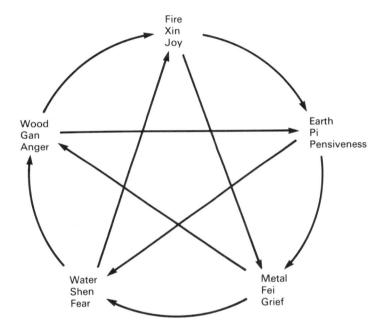

In Five Phase Theory, there are set correspondences between Phases, Zang and emotions, as shown in Figure 15.1. It is said that via the cycle of Sheng, (Promotion or Production), each emotion may give rise to the next by the 'Mother-Son' relationship, for example, fear promotes anger. Also, via the cycle of Ko (Control or Conquest), each restrains and is itself restrained. For example, fear controls joy, and joy controls grief. A third relationship is that within each Phase, an excess of the emotion may injure the Zang, or conversely, may result from disharmony of that Zang. For example, excess anger injures Gan, or Gan disharmony may be associated with excess anger.

However, anger, for example, does not always give rise to joy, nor does joy always arise from anger. Also, pensiveness may control emotions other than fear, and fear may be controlled by emotions other than pensiveness. Again, excess grief may not injure Fei, Fei disharmony may not be accompanied by grief, grief may injure Zang other than Fei, and Fei may be injured by emotions other than grief.

In general, the Five Phase Theory approach to the emotions is incomplete, limited, rigid and artificial. It is only of use in giving a preliminary, theoretical understanding of emotional relationships, and its use in the clinic all too often leads to the facts being twisted to suit the theory, rather than the theory being adjusted to suit the facts. The variety of human emotion is subtle and complex, and ill-suited to the restrictions of a rigid system of classification.

Emotions and Yin Yang

Lack of any emotion, whether from obstruction or Deficiency, may be seen as Yin, whereas excess of any emotion may be seen as Yang. However, some emotions seem more Yin or more Yang than others; for example anger is more Yang and active than pensiveness, and joy may be more Yang and extrovert than sorrow and anxiety.

Nevertheless, each emotion has its own Yin and Yang aspects, which may transform into each other:- frustration may rise up as anger, and fall back into depression; fear has its more Yin, passive aspects of paralysis and immobility, which may transform into its more Yang aspects of flight and fight.

The arbitrary division of people into Deficient Yin and Deficient Yang types, discussed on page 204, may include emotions. The thinner, Deficient Yin type tends to irritability, anger, restlessness, hypersensitivity and extroversion; whilst the plumper, Deficient Yang type tends to be more phlegmatic, less active, and more introvert and prone to depression. However, this is a gross over-simplification, and of use only as a most general guideline.

More specifically, Deficient Shen Yin, the foundation of Deficient Yin of the other Zang, is associated with signs of Heat and anxiety, whilst Deficient Shen Yang is more associated with signs of Cold and depression. If Yin Deficiency includes Deficient Xin Yin, there may be Disturbance of Shen*, with over-excitement and irritability. If Yang Deficiency includes Deficient Xin Yang and Deficient Xin Qi, there may be Deficiency of Shen*, with dullness and lack of joy and vitality. If Xin is obstructed by Phlegm, there may be a predominantly Yin pattern, Cold Phlegm Misting Xin, with signs more of introversion, depression and inactivity; or there may be a predominantly Yang pattern, Phlegm Fire Agitating Xin, with signs more of extroversion, violent mania, and hyperactivity.

Emotions and Substances

Deficiency of the Substances may be arranged into two groups with respect to the emotions:-

Deficient Yang Group	Deficient Yin Group
Deficient Qi	Deficient Xue
Deficient Shen*	Disturbance of Shen*
Deficient Jing	Deficient Jin Ye

The Deficient Yang group may be associated with introversion, depression, lack of joy, and general dull emotional response; and the Deficient Yin group may be associated with extroversion, anxiety, mania, and general emotional excess. However, this is only a very general guideline, since there is much overlap between the Substances and their Disharmonies, as discussed in Chapter 3, and since there are several facets to each Substance. For example in the case of Xue, there are various aspects and various factors involved, as shown in Table 15.3.

Stagnation, Phlegm, and Internal Wind, are all associated with obstruction or irregularity in the flow of Qi and Xue, and may involve emotional disharmony of both Yin and Yang types. This is considered in greater detail in other chapters.

Table 15.3 Disharmonies of Xue and Emotions

Aspect of Xue	Zang Fu Disharmonies	Emotional Disharmonies
Formation of Xue	Deficient Qi and Yang of Pi and Wei	pensiveness & worry
	Deficient Shen Jing	fear & fright
Movement of Xue	Deficient Yang of Shen, Xin and Fei	fear & fright sadness & grief
Evenness of Movement of Xue	Depression of Gan Qi	irritation, anger, frustration, depression
Holding of Xue in Xue Mai	Deficient Qi and Yang of Pi Heat in Gan Xue	pensiveness, worry anger, irritation, frustration

Emotions and Jing Luo

Basically, Jing Luo may suffer from four main problems:-

Deficiency of Qi and Xue
Obstruction of Flow of Qi and Xue
Irregularity or Disturbance of Flow of Qi and Xue
Presence of Disease Factor

In practice, there is often overlap between these four closely related problems. For example, obstruction in the flow of Qi and Xue may result in temporary Deficiency of Qi and Xue in front of the obstruction, and temporary Excess of Qi and Xue behind it. Conversely, Deficiency may give rise to Stagnation of Qi and Xue. Also, obstruction may be closely linked with irregularity, disturbance and fluctuation in the flow of Substances through Jing Luo. Rebellious Qi, i.e. Qi moving in an inappropriate direction, is a particular case of irregularity of Qi flow. The fourth category of presence of Disease Factor, may include both External and Internal types of Wind, Cold, Heat, Damp and Dryness; and also Phlegm.

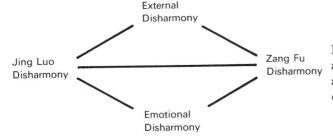

Emotional disharmony may give rise to any combination of these four categories, and vice versa; linking External Factors, emotional factors, Zang Fu and Jing Luo.

Mental Faculties and Emotions

The distinction made here between the feelings or emotions, and the intellectual faculties or mental abilities, is rather arbitrary, since the two are inextricably interlinked. However, the 'Nei Jing' associated specific intellectual faculties with certain of the Zang Fu, often in terms of officials of State:-

Xin is the Sovereign Ruler who directs with clear insight; Fei is the Minister in charge of rhythmic order; Gan is the General who excels through his strategic planning, whilst Dan is the Official who excels through his decisions and judgment; Pi is the repository of imagination and ideas; whilst Shen stores the willpower and is associated with technical skills, excelling through his ability and cleverness.

Table 15.4 links the Five Zang with their respective mental faculties, but there is considerable vagueness and overlap. For example, clear thinking may be linked with Shen, in terms of mental skill and cleverness; with Pi in terms of clear manipulation and storage of ideas; with Gan, in terms of the balanced expression of those ideas; and with Xin, in terms of clear, directed consciousness.

Table 15.4 The Five Zang and the Mental Faculties

Zang	Faculty
Shen	Stores and governs the Will
Pi	Stores and governs the imagination, ideas and memory
Gan	Residence of Hun, Soul; governs emotions, mental balance and conduct
Xin	Residence of Shen*, Spirit, mind; governs consciousness, clear thinking and insight
Fei	Residence of Po, Animal Spirit; governs sensations and movement

Whilst the faculties are listed, they are not given the same importance as physical or emotional factors, and are rarely listed as either origins or signs of Zang Fu disharmony.

Clinical Importance of Emotional Disharmony

There are two main aspects of the Clinical Importance of the Emotions:-
   (i) As factors originating Zang Fu disharmony
   (ii) As signs of Zang Fu disharmony

Chapters 7 to 11 on the five Zang give outline diagrams of the origins of disharmony of each Zang, and also give lists of the signs of disharmony characteristic of each of these organ systems.

In the case of Gan, anger, irritation, frustration and depression may all contribute to the patterns of Gan disharmony. These emotions, along with hypersensitivity and the tendency to overreact to environmental stimuli, are also signs characteristic of Gan imbalance.

In the case of Xin, however, excess Joy is not generally listed as either a sign or an originating factor of Xin disharmony. Precipitating factors of Xin imbalance disharmony may include anxiety, mental irritation, depression, sadness and grief. Anxiety and mental irritation may lead to Disturbance of Shen*, and depression, sadness and grief may result in Stagnation of Qi and Xue, perhaps with eventual production of Fire and Phlegm. The mental irritation associated with Xin is perhaps more linked with sensations of anxiety and panic, than the mental irritation associated with Gan, which is perhaps more concerned with anger and irritability. Similarly, the Xin type depression is perhaps more linked with sadness and melancholy, than the Gan type depression linked with frustration. However, mental irritation and depression can affect both Xin and Gan, and which is predominantly affected will depend on the predisposition of the individual and on the situation at the particular time. Indeed, both Zang may be affected by depression and irritability at the same time, so that signs of both Xin and Gan disharmony are manifested. Signs of Deficient Shen* may include apathy and lack of joie de vivre, and depressive, introverted behaviour, whereas signs of Disturbed Shen* include restlessness, anxiety, fearfulness and irritability, or, in extreme cases, insanity and violent behaviour.

Fear and fright are listed as factors that may originate Shen disorders, but are not often listed as signs of Shen disharmony. Similarly, excess thinking or preoccupied thinking, i.e. worry, may be factors in Pi imbalance, but are not usually listed as important signs of Pi disharmony. Grief is listed as neither origin or sign of Fei imbalance. Indeed, Gan and Xin are the two Zang most affected by the Stagnation of Qi associated with grief.

In summary, Gan and Xin are the two Zang for which emotional factors are most important in precipitating disease, but anger and joy are not the only emotions involved here; and, in the case of Xin, joy may not be the only, or even the main, emotional sign of Xin disharmony. Fear and preoccupation may injure Shen and Pi respectively, but are not listed as main signs in the disharmony pattern of these organ systems. The origins and signs listed for Fei disharmony do not generally include grief.

However, just because an emotion is not generally listed as an originating factor or as a sign of Zang disharmony, does not mean that it is unimportant in this context. It simply means that some Chinese texts consider other factors or signs of greater clinical relevance.

Treatment of Emotional Disharmony

Diagnosis, treatment, and patient education, in cases involving emotional disharmony, are according to the usual principles; and choice of points and methods of point use will depend on the situation of the particular patient.

Cases involving emotional disharmony may be arbitrarily divided into two types:-

General Cases
Cases of Severe Mental Illness

The category of general cases, includes those patients where emotional disharmony is an important component of the Pattern of Disharmony, whether emotional disharmony is the presenting sign or not.

This category includes a large proportion of all patients coming for treatment, since emotional and mental stress are involved in almost every case to some degree, as discussed elsewhere (20).

The category of severe mental illness is represented by far fewer patients in general acupuncture practice, since patients suffering from extreme emotional and mental imbalance are often not capable of normal functioning, and are confined in specialist hospitals. Whereas patients in the general category may come to the surgery for treatment once a week or once a month, in the average situation, patients suffering from severe mental illness generally need to be treated in hospital or home situation on a more or less daily basis.

However, in practice, there is no sharp distinction between the two categories, and indeed a person may suffer from chronic, moderate emotional disharmony with periodic acute severe crises. Whereas acupuncture can be very effective in most general cases, results in cases of severe mental illness can be very slow, and there may be a strong tendency to relapse. Nevertheless, research is being carried out in China on the treatment of severe mental illnesses by TCM, and progress is being made.

Examples of cases involving general emotional disharmony are given throughout this book, and some details of severe mental illness are given in the next section.

Treatment of Severe Mental Illness

General Principles

The general aim of treatment is to disperse Hyperactive Yang, Blazing Fire, Stirring of Internal Wind and Phlegm, to regulate Qi, and to calm the mind and clear the Brain. Since Yang, Fire, and Wind tend to rise and obstruct the channels of the head, points on the head are important here. Points on the limbs, especially below the knees and elbows, and especially from Shen, Xin, Xin Bao and Gan channels, may be used as secondary points.

Reinforcing, reducing or even methods of needle manipulation, may be used as appropriate, in some cases with moxa or with electro-stimulation.

Examples of Head Points

Frontal Region

Shenting	Du 24	Calms mind and promotes clear thinking and memory.
Meichong	BL.3	Helps disorders arising from upward disturbance of Qi and hence sensory and perceptual problems.
Toulinqi	GB.15	Apoplectic coma, emotional disturbance.
Benshen	GB.13	Gathers Qi together, preventing it from splitting up. (These four points all treat seizures and vertigo).

Parietal Region

Houding	Du 19	Disturbances of perception.
Baihui	Du 20	Disturbances of perception and movement.
Qianding	Du 21	Excessive movement and speaking.
Xuanlu	GB.5	Disturbances of speech.

Temporal Region

Shuaigu	GB.8	Deafness and auditory hallucination.
Tianchong	GB.9	Disturbance of hearing.
Yifeng	TB.17	Auditory hallucination, ringing sound in brain.
Luxi	TB.19	

Occipital Region

Fengchi	GB.20	Optic atrophy.
Tianzhu	BL.10	Ataxia.

Examples of Point Combinations

Coma

First group	Baihui, Du 20; Yintang, M-HN-3; Daling, P.7
Second group	Benshen, GB.13; Shenting, Du 24; Renzhong, Du 26
	(Treat every day, alternating first and second group)

Dreamy State

First group	Dazhui, Du 14; Yanglingquan, GB.34
Second group	Shenque, Ren 8; Guanyuan, Ren 4
	(If the second group is selected, mild moxa can be used)

Disturbance of Thinking

First group	Baihui, Du 20; Luoque, BL.8; Tongli, HE. 5; Dazhong, KID. 4
Second group	Baihui, Du 20; Fengchi, GB.20; Shenmen, HE. 7; Taixi, KID. 3
	(These point combinations are used where thinking is interrupted, so that, for example, the patient cannot finish a sentence)

Conditions of mania and depression, associated with Xin disharmony, are discussed on page 112; and patterns involving violent aggressive behaviour are discussed on page 133, under Gan Disharmony.

Examples of Case Histories
The following two brief case histories are of patients treated in a Nanjing mental hospital in 1981.
1. An adult male schizophrenic, had the pattern of wanting to eat his stool and urine, and of wanting to die. Treatment with Western medicine was unsatisfactory.

Acupuncture using head points, and Chinese herbal medicine were used, and the patient was much improved after 6 months treatment. The needles were retained for 1 hour each treatment, and the main points used were:-

Shangxing,   Du 23, through to Shenting,   Du 24
Touwei,   ST. 8, through to Benshen,   GB.13
Houding,   Du 19, through to Tianchong,   GB. 9

2.   An adult male suffered from various fantasies, for example he imagined himself to be the heroes of various films, and thought his doctor was his father. Western medicine was used in conjunction with acupuncture and the following points were used:-

Baihui, Du 20; Qianding, Du 21; Touwei, ST. 8; and Ermen, TB.21, through Tinggong, SI.19, to Tinghui, GB.2.

Summary

The interrelationship of emotions and Zang Fu patterns of disharmony is of supreme clinical importance. In the West, most illness is originated by, aggravated by, or associated with emotional disturbance.

Although the terminology of the Seven Emotions and the Five Feelings is too limited to represent properly the full range of human emotions, acupuncture treatment can help greatly in a very wide range of general cases involving emotional disharmony.

In the field of severe mental illness, especially where patients are confined to home or hospital, the result of acupuncture treatment may be slower and less marked. However, research is being carried out, and, at least in some cases, some degree of relief may be obtained. Usually, the patients are treated in the hospital situation, every day, or every other day.

Chapter
16

Disharmonies Involving More than One Zang

Disharmonies of Two Zang Together

This section investigates the commonly occuring Patterns of Disharmony involving two Zang together.

Xin and Fei:- Deficient Qi of Xin and Fei
Xin and Fei are intimately associated in two main functions:-

Formation of Qi and Xue
Movement of Qi and Xue

Formation of Qi and Xue
Both Xin and Fei are involved in the formation of Qi and Xue in the chest, as discussed in Chapter 3, and summarized in Figure 16.1.

Figure 16.1 Formation of Qi and Xue

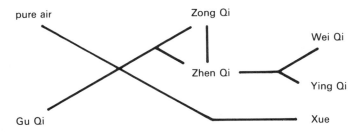

Movement of Qi and Xue

Zong Qi, the Qi of the Chest, gathers in the chest, forming the Sea of Qi. It regulates the movements of heartbeat and respiration, and assists Fei and Xin respectively, in the movement of Qi and of Xue throughout the Body. Hence, via Zong Qi, Xin and Fei are intimately related, both in health and in disease. Deficiencies of Qi, of Xin and of Fei often occur together, with the simultaneous occurrence of such signs as palpitation and shortness of breath. Via Zong Qi, factors tending to weaken Xin will tend to weaken Fei, and vice versa. Also, via Zong Qi, various factors tend to weaken Xin and Fei simultaneously. Some of these are outlined in Table 16.1, along with appropriate remedial actions.

Signs

Deficiency of Qi of Xin and Fei may occur, for example, in chronic cardiac insufficiency with bronchitis, and signs may include:- palpitations, spontaneous perspiration, shortness of breath, asthma, weak cough, weak or frail pulse, pale tongue.

Table 16.1 Zong Qi, Fei and Xin

Disease Factors	Remedy
poor posture & breathing	correct posture, breathing exercises
contaminated air	wear mask, adjust working conditions
smoking	stop smoking
External Cold lack of exercise	keep warm sufficient, appropriate exercise
chest injury	appropriate treatment & remedial exercises
emotional disturbances	support, counselling, treatment, time

Xin and Pi:- Deficient Xin Xue and Deficient Pi Qi

If Pi Qi is Deficient, and fails to produce sufficient Xue, Deficiency of Xin Xue may result, with involvement of signs of Deficiency of both Xin Xue and Pi Qi, as in some forms of anaemia, insomnia and cardiac insufficiency.

Signs

Signs may include:- palpitations, dull pale complexion, insomnia, lethargy, poor appetite, loose stools, weak or thin pulse, pale tongue.

Xin and Shen:- Deficient Yang of both Xin and Shen

Xin Yang Deficiency may occur with Deficient Shen Yang, or may be originated or aggravated by it. This combination may progress to Stagnant Xin Xue, Collapse of Xin Yang, or to additional involvement of Fei, with Water Radiating to Fei. This combination may be seen in certain cases of cardiac insufficiency.

Signs

Signs may include:- palpitation, feelings of cold, oedema of limbs, face and eyelids, scanty urine, frail, minute, knotted or intermittent pulse, and pale flabby moist tongue, with white coat.

Xin and Shen:- Xin and Shen Not Harmonious

The balance of Fire and Water, Xin and Shen, may be looked at in terms of the polarity of Yin and Yang within each Zang, so that each has its Fire and Water aspect:-

Figure 16.2 Yin and Yang, Xin and Shen

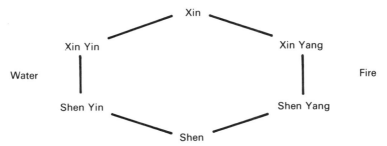

Alternatively, the relationship of 'Mutual Support of Fire and Water', 'Mutual Support of Xin and Shen', may be seen in terms of a polarity where Shen is predominantly Water, and Xin is predominantly Fire, each supporting the other:-

Figure 16.3 Fire and Water, Xin and Shen

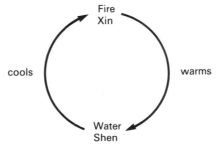

If these Yin - Yang, Fire - Water relationships are balanced, Xin and Shen are in harmony. If, for example, Shen Yin is Deficient, then it cannot control and cool Xin Fire, which then flares up, with signs such as insomnia and irritability. In such a case where both Shen and Xin Yin are Deficient, Xin and Shen are said to 'Lose Communication', as in certain cases of insomnia.

Signs

Signs may include:- palpitation, irritability, insomnia, dry throat, night sweats, lumbago, thin rapid pulse, and red dry tongue with little coat.

Xin and Gan:- Deficient Yin of Xin and Gan
Xin and Gan are the two Zang Fu most concerned with the maintenance of emotional harmony.

Figure 16.4 Gan, Xin and Depression

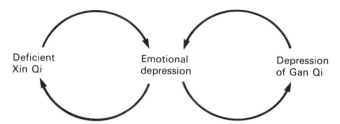

Emotional disharmony may give rise to disharmony of Xin or Gan or vice versa, whether the emotional disharmony is depression or mental irritation:-

Figure 16.5 Xin, Gan and Mental Irritation

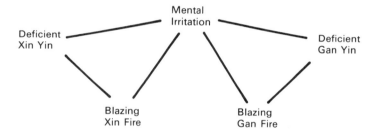

Since mental irritation may originate Deficient Yin of both Xin and Gan, these two patterns often occur together, often in combination with Deficient Shen Yin, as in certain cases of insomnia or menopausal problems. In more extreme cases, severe anxiety, depression and anger may give rise to Blazing Fire of Xin and Gan, which rises up the Body, accompanied by Phlegm, and obstructs and disturbs Shen★, with signs of violent insanity.

Signs
Signs may include:- restlessness, excitability, irritability, insomnia, headache, night sweats, wiry thin and rapid pulse, and red tongue, especially at tip, and with red dots on the sides, which is dry with little coat.

Shen and Gan:- Deficient Yin of Shen and Gan
This combination is a common forerunner and associate of the previous combination. If Shen Yin is Deficient, then Gan Yin will not be properly nourished, and Gan Yang will not be properly controlled as in Hyperactive Gan Yang. Also, Yin may not properly control Fire, resulting in Blazing Gan Fire. Both Hyperactive Gan Yang and Blazing Gan Fire may lead to Stirring of Gan Wind. Hence, Deficient Shen Yin may allow Gan Yang, Fire and Wind to rebel

upwards, combining with Phlegm, to disrupt and obstruct the Qi in the channels of the head, and confuse the mind and Senses. This is seen, for example, in epilepsy or CVA. This combination of Deficient Yin of Shen and Gan may also occur in chronic glomerular nephritis, abnormal uterine bleeding, and amenorrhoea.

Signs
Signs may include:- headache, vertigo, anger, insomnia, red cheeks, hot palms and soles, painful flanks, sore back, perhaps hemiplegia, wiry thin and rapid pulse, and red tongue with little coat.

There is a less important pattern of **Deficient Xin Qi and Deficient Dan Qi**, with signs of insomnia, timidity, dream-disturbed sleep, tendency to waken in fright, wiry thin pulse, and pale tongue. This pattern combines the fearfulness of Deficient Xin Qi with the timidity and lack of confidence of Deficient Dan Qi. This combination is seen in certain cases of insomnia.

Gan and Pi:- Gan Invades Pi
There is a close relationship between the Free-flowing function of Gan, and the Transforming and Transporting functions of Pi. If the Free-flowing function of Gan becomes impaired, Depression of Gan Qi, and the associated retardation and stagnation of Qi flow, tend to depress the digestive function of Pi and Wei. Although this is termed Gan Invading Pi, Dan and Wei may also be involved. There may also be the additional associations of Blazing Gan Fire and Blazing Wei Fire, and of Damp Heat in Gan and Dan, and Damp Heat accumulating in Pi, depending on the circumstances.

If Pi is Deficient, then Gan is more likely to invade, hence the headaches and irritability that accompany hunger in some individuals, that are reduced after eating. This pattern is seen in various cases of indigestion, vomiting, diarrhoea and abdominal pain.

Signs
Signs include:- irritability, moodiness, soreness and distension of chest and flanks, nausea, vomiting, abdominal pain and discomfort, flatulence, loss of appetite, loose stools, wiry pulse, and dark or normal tongue with white coat.

Pi and Shen:- Deficient Pi Qi and Deficient Shen Yang
Shen is responsible for the prenatal constitution, Pi is responsible for the postnatal constitution. Shen Jing is needed to activate digestion, and the process of digestion is required to supplement the replenishable postnatal aspect of Jing. One of the important functions of Chong Mai is that by connecting Shen with Pi, it links Prenatal (Congenital) Qi to Postnatal (Acquired) Qi, and hence is clinically useful in cases of weak digestion linked to poor constitution. The Transforming and Transporting functions of Pi depend on Pi Yang, and hence on Shen Yang, for warming, activation and movement.

If Wei and Pi Yang are Deficient, the Transforming and Transporting functions of Pi will be impaired, Qi and Xue formation will be deficient, Jin Ye will not be properly metabolised, and turbid Jin Ye will accumulate with formation of oedema and Phlegm.

This pattern is seen in various cases of oedema, diarrhoea, anaemia, pelvic inflammatory disease, and acute glomerulo-nephritis.

Signs

Signs may include:- cold limbs, cold, sore lower back, oedema, difficult urination, perhaps clear leukorrhoea, loose stools with undigested food, weak deep pulse, and pale flabby moist tongue with white coat.

Pi and Fei:- Deficient Pi Qi and Deficient Fei Qi

Pi and Fei are linked in the formation and movement of Qi, Xue and Jin Ye. Pi sends Gu Qi up to the chest where, under the influence of Xin and Fei, Zong Qi, Zhen Qi and Xue are formed. Also, Pi sends up the pure fraction of the fluids to Fei as vapour; Fei is involved in the formation of Qi and Jin Ye, and is responsible for their proper distribution throughout the Body.

If Pi Qi is Deficient, then Fei Qi, which depends on Gu Qi to nourish Zong Qi and Zhen Qi in the chest, will tend to become Deficient. Also, it is said that Pi forms Phlegm and Fei stores it. If Phlegm forms, due to weakness of the ability of Pi to Transform and to Transport Jin Ye, Phlegm may accumulate in Fei, if Fei Qi is Deficient, and the Dispersing power of Fei is weak. Furthermore, Damp tends to accumulate if Pi Qi is Deficient, and if Fei cannot properly perform its Descending function of sending fluid down to Shen, oedema may develop.

This pattern is seen in certain cases of convalescence, malnutrition and oedema.

Signs

Signs may include:- lack of energy, loss of appetite, shortness of breath, cough, asthma, copious thin white phlegm, loose stools, oedema, weak pulse, and pale tongue with white coat.

Fei and Shen:- Deficient Fei Qi and Deficient Shen Yang

This combination is known as 'Shen Unable to Grasp Qi'. The Descending function of Fei is responsible for sending Qi down to Shen; Shen is responsible for receiving and holding the Qi. If Shen Qi and Yang are weak, and Shen does not properly grasp the Qi, it rebels upwards, impairing the Fei function of respiration, resulting in asthma.

In addition, if Shen Yang is Deficient, the actions of Shen, Pi and Fei in transforming and circulating Jin Ye will be impaired, Fei will not properly send liquids down to Shen, nor Shen send vapour up to Fei. This will result in accumulation of Damp, oedema and urinary problems.

Alternatively, Shen Yin may not properly nourish Fei Yin, and if Fei Yin is Deficient, Fei may become dry, hot and inflamed, as in the Deficient Yin form of pulmonary tuberculosis, or the Fire form of diabetes mellitus.

Signs

Signs may include:- asthma, difficult inhalation, shortness of breath aggravated by exertion, spontaneous sweating, cold limbs, low voice, listlessness, weak or frail pulse, and pale flabby moist tongue.

Gan and Fei:- Gan Fire Invades Fei

Blazing of Gan Fire may flare upwards and affect the Descending function of Fei, causing coughing; and the Dispersing function of Fei, causing Dryness. Also, the Heat may cause Xue to leak from Xue Mai, so that there may be coughing of blood.

Signs

Signs may include:- irritability and anger, burning pain in chest and flank, dry throat, coughing blood or phlegm with blood, red eyes, bitter taste, dark urine, constipation, wiry rapid pulse, and red tongue with thin dry yellow coat.

In addition, there is the relationship between Gan and Fei based on the Fei function of governing movement of Qi, and the Gan function of Free- flowing of Qi. Hence, both Gan and Fei are affected by emotional depression, sadness, melancholy and grief; with the associated depression of movement of Qi, and Stagnation of Qi in the chest. In the case of Gan, Depression of Qi would be more associated with depression, frustration, irritation; frequent sighing, digestive and menstrual problems. In the case of Fei, depression of Qi would be more associated with grief, melancholy, sadness, lack of Shen, weak voice, sobbing, restricted breathing, and Qi Deficiency as well as Stagnation. The predominant pattern would depend on the emotional predisposition of the individual and on the circumstances.

Disharmonies of Three or More Zang Together

Only a few of the common combinations of three or more Zang will be considered, since this section quickly develops into the next stage:- the study of Common Disease Patterns. The basis of the groups of three or more Zang together is the division into Deficient Yin and Deficient Yang.

Deficient Yin Group

Any combination of Deficient Shen, Gan, Xin, Fei and Wei may occur, and the combinations of Gan and Xin, and of Gan and Fei, mentioned in the previous section, often include Shen:-

Deficient Yin of Shen, Gan and Xin
Deficient Yin of Shen, Gan and Fei

Deficient Yang Group

It is possible to find any combination of Deficient Yang of Shen, Pi, Xin, Fei and Wei. The difference between the Deficient Yang and the Deficient Yin lists is that the former contains Pi, but not Gan, and the latter contains Gan but not Pi. This results from the natures of Pi and of Gan, the former is susceptible to Damp and Deficient Yang, and the latter to Dryness and Deficient Yin.

Certain combinations that have already had brief mention are:-

Deficient Yang of Shen, Pi and Xin
Deficient Yang of Shen, Pi and Fei
Deficient Yang of Shen, Pi and Wei

Shen, Pi and Xin

The combination of Deficient Yang of Shen and Pi is likely to accompany such Xin disharmonies as Deficient Xin Yang, Stagnant Xin Xue, and Misting of Xin by Cold Phlegm. The foundation of the Deficient Yang of Pi and Xin is Deficient Shen Yang. Poor Transformation and Transportation of Pi leads to accumulation of Phlegm. In conditions of Deficient Xin Qi and Yang, where the circulation of

Qi and Xue in Xin is impaired, Phlegm may become involved in the pattern of retardation and stagnation of movement. This may give rise to feelings of stuffiness in the chest, and lethargy, or, in more severe cases, to speech defects, mental confusion or loss of consciousness.

Shen, Pi and Fei

These are the three main Zang Fu involved in Jin Ye metabolism and the cycle of Jin Ye circulation (see pages 69 and 84). If Yang, the aspect that warms, activates, transforms and moves, is Deficient, then Jin Ye metabolism and circulation will be defective. If Shen Yang is Deficient, Shen cannot properly vaporise the fluid and send it up to Fei, nor properly drive the processes of separation, absorption and transformation of Jin Ye that occur in Xiao Chang, Da Chang and Pang Guang. Also, Shen will be unable properly to assist the processes of digestion in Pi and Wei, and the Dispersing and Descending carried out by the Yang aspect of Fei Qi. Deficient Yang of Pi means improper Transformation and Transportation of food and drink, tending to result in Deficiency of Qi and Xue, and also in accumulation of turbid Jin Ye, Damp and perhaps Phlegm. Deficient Yang of Fei means poor Dispersing and Descending functions of Fei, so that fluid is not properly moved and sent down to Shen, with resulting oedema and perhaps accumulation of Phlegm or fluid in Fei.

Shen, Pi and Wei

Deficient Yang of Shen may be associated with Deficient Yang of both Pi and Wei, leading to poor digestion, and facilitating Invasion by External Cold and Damp, or accumulation of Internal Cold and Damp, with retention of partly digested food in Wei, and the presence of undigested food in the stools. This combination is discussed in greater detail below, under Digestive Problems.

Emotional Disharmonies

Various groups of combinations are possible here, indeed the emotions continually fluctuate and change in the interaction of the individual and the environment. However, two commonly occuring groups are:-

Deficient Yin of Shen, Gan and Xin
Depression of Function of Gan, Xin and Fei

Deficient Yin of Shen, Gan and Xin

This has been listed under the Deficient Yin group above, and is commonly associated with the emotional patterns of anxiety, restlessness, irritability, over-excitability, hypersensitivity and overreaction to environmental stimuli. It is seen in many Patterns of Disharmony, including insomnia, hypertension, certain menopausal neuroses and hyperactivity, and, in extreme forms, when it has developed into patterns of Blazing Fire accompanied by Phlegm and Wind, it may be a part of such diseases as CVA and many forms of insanity.

Depression of Function of Gan, Xin and Fei

The relationship of Gan and Fei in this context has already been discussed (see page 201). Emotions such as melancholy, sadness and grief, are likely to affect Xin as well as Fei, since they will depress the functions of Zong Qi. Depression of Gan, Xin and Fei may occur together. If Depression of Gan Qi is predominant, there may be depression, frustration, anger and a predominance of Gan signs. If Deficient Xin Qi predominates, there may be signs of Deficient Shen*, such as lack of joy, apathy, and mental and emotional dullness. If Fei functions are depressed, there may be weak voice, restricted breathing, and possibly manifestations of grief. In the case of Xin and Gan, moods of depression and introversion may alternate with moods of hyperactivity, excess talking or outbursts of anger. In extreme cases, there may be fluctuations between violent mania and extreme depression. These alternations may represent fluctuations in the movement of Qi and the emotions, associated with temporary obstruction followed by temporary clearing of the blockage, before the obstruction builds up again. Alternatively, there may be chronic Stagnation of Qi, and emotions, which eventually and periodically give rise to Fire, which blazes upwards. In more extreme cases, for example obstruction and disturbance of Xin by Phlegm, the presence of Phlegm obstructing the Orifices of Xin Senses, may result in more severe symptoms.

Digestive Problems

The main three Zang Fu involved in digestive disorders are Pi, Wei and Gan. In addition, Dan, Xiao Chang and Da Chang are involved, but are of lesser importance, and Xiao Chang and Da Chang are generally treated with points from Pi or Wei channels. The interactions between Pi, Wei and Gan, Yin and Yang, Cold and Heat are summarised in Figure 16.6.

The basic division in this diagram is into Deficient Yin and Deficient Yang. Shen and Wei have patterns of both Deficient Yin and Deficient Yang, and are therefore at the centre of the diagram. Gan tends to Deficient Yin and not to Deficient Yang, and Pi tends to Deficient Yang and not to Deficient Yin. Thus, while Shen and Wei may be affected by both External Heat and External Cold, Gan is predominantly affected by External Heat, since it already tends to Heat and Dryness, and Pi is predominantly affected by External Cold and Damp, since it inherently tends to Coldness and Damp. Gan may also be affected by Cold, as Stagnation of Cold in Gan Jing Luo, and Pi may have patterns associated with Heat, for example Damp Heat accumulates in Pi, but these patterns are not the predominant ones.

Wei has patterns of Deficient Yin and Blazing Fire like Gan, but also those of Deficient Yang and Invasion by Cold, like Pi. Also, along with Pi, it may be Invaded by Gan, during Depression of Gan Qi, especially if Pi and Wei Qi are Deficient.

Figure 16.6 also divides people into two types; the Yin Deficient Type and the Yang Deficient Type. Obviously, this is a gross generalisation, but it is nevertheless a most interesting one. The Yin Deficient type tends to have a thin face and wiry body; with quick, nervous, restless, edgy mannerisms and movements. Such people may be prone to physical, mental and sexual hyperactivity, irritability and insomnia; if male, to premature ejaculation, and if female, to premenstrual irritability and menopausal flushing. The Yang Deficient type tends to be plump of face and body, due to accumulation of Phlegm, and more placid, with slower movements. This type tends to hypoactivity, dullness and hypersomnia, with less sexual interest, and, if male, tend to be slower to get an

Figure 16.6 Interrelationships of Pi, Wei and Gan, Yin and Yang, Cold and Heat

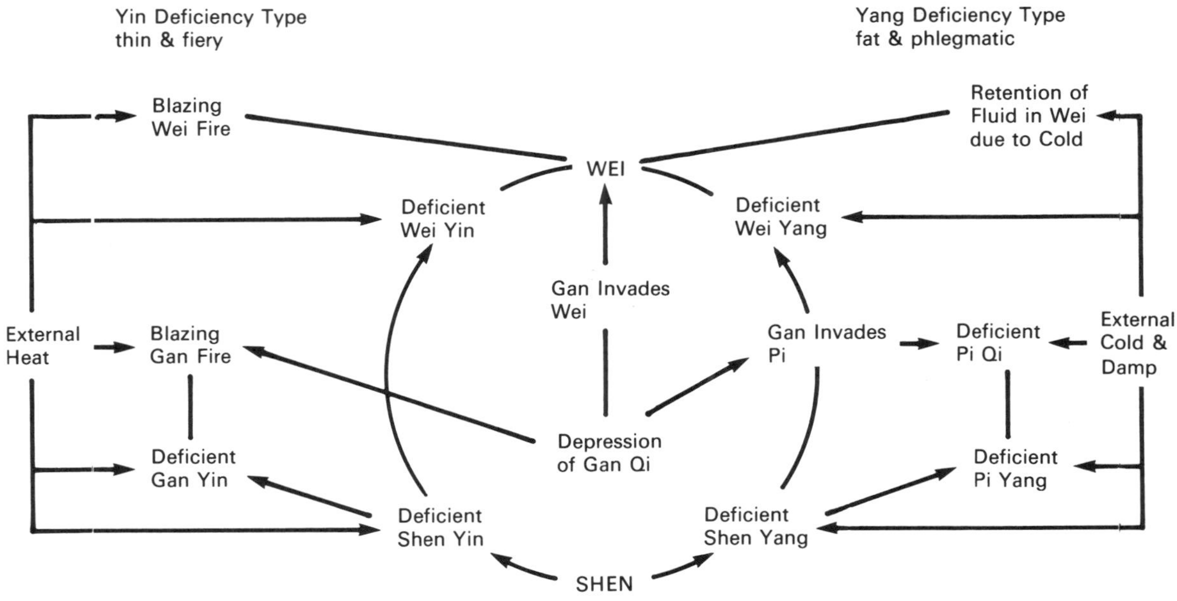

Yin Deficiency Type
thin & fiery

Yang Deficiency Type
fat & phlegmatic

erection, and if female, to premenstrual and menopausal depression. In the Yin
Deficient type, the pulse tends to be thin rapid and wiry; with thin red tongue.
The Yang Deficient type tends to have slower, deeper, slippery pulse; with fuller,
moister, paler tongue, with thicker greasy white coat.

One manifestation of the difference between the two types is in appetite for food.
The Yin Deficient type will tend to be hungry more frequently, with sensations of
irritability, light-headedness or headaches. This is due to the reciprocal relationship
between Gan and Pi, whereby, in this case, an empty stomach represents temporary
Deficiency of Pi and Wei Qi, so that Gan can more readily invade Pi and Wei. Also,
Hyperactive Gan Yang rises to the head, causing signs of light-headedness, headache
and irritability. The Yang Deficient type may eat frequently due to depression or
boredom, but does not suffer from feelings of hunger in the same way as the Yin
Deficient type, and is more prone to gain weight, partly since the Yang Deficiency
results in poor Transformation and Transportation by Pi, with accumulation of
Phlegm, and partly since this type of person is usually less active than the Yin
Deficient type. Also, Yin Deficient people tend to drink larger amounts of colder
drinks than Yang Deficient individuals, who prefer lesser volumes of warmer drinks.
For example, in a pub, an individual tending to Yin Deficiency might ask for a pint
of cold lager, since Yin Deficiency tends to be associated with Heat and Dryness;
whereas a Yang Deficient individual might ask for a whisky, since Yang Deficiency
tends to Cold and Damp, so that this type would avoid excess volume and choose a
drink that would 'warm them up'.

However, although these general tendencies exist, and are important in
differential diagnosis, the situation in clinical practice is rarely so simple and clear-
cut. An individual may manifest signs of both Deficient Yin and Deficient Yang
simultaneously; or may show Deficient Yin signs on one occasion, and Deficient

Yang signs on another; or some Zang Fu may have patterns of Yin Deficiency, whilst at the same time other Zang Fu in the same individual may have patterns of Deficient Yang; as described on page 23.

Gynaecological and Obstetric Disorders

Physiology

The three main Zang involved in the physiology and pathology of gynaecology and obstetrics are Shen, Pi and Gan. Shen is directly linked to the uterus, and to Chong Mai and Ren Mai. Pi and Gan communicate with the uterus via the Rhen Mai and Chong Mai.

Figure 16.7 Zang Fu Interrelationships in Gynaecology & Obstetrics

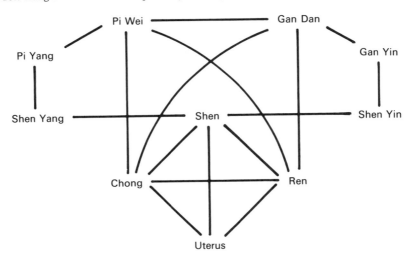

Figure 16.7 shows the main relationships involved in mensturation and gestation. These processes depend especially on an adequate supply of Xue, and this depends on the proper functioning of a number of Zang Fu and Jing Luo.

Xue

Pi, Wei, Xin, Fei and Shen are involved in various capacities, in the formation of Xue. Gan and Chong Mai are concerned with storage of Xue, and Gan and Pi are responsible for holding Xue in Xue Mai. Xin rules the circulation of Xue, Gan is responsible for its smooth and even movement, and Chong Mai and Ren Mai are also concerned in ensuring that this movement is free and unobstructed, especially in the lower abdomen. Also, if Fei is Deficient, Qi may become Deficient, and since Qi moves Xue, the circulation of Xue may be weakened.

Pathology

The interactions of the Zang Fu and the Disease Factors will now be considered in the origin of the gynaecological and obstetric disorders. The three main Zang Fu involved are Shen, Pi and Gan.

Shen

Deficient Shen Yin and Deficient Shen Yang, the foundations for Deficient Yin or Deficient Yang of the other Zang Fu, originate as follows:-

Figure 16.8 Origins of Shen Disharmonies

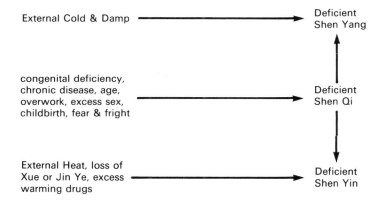

Pi

Just as Shen is the foundation of Congenital Qi, Pi is the foundation of Acquired Qi in the Body. Pi disharmony may originate as follows:-

Figure 16.9 Origins of Pi Disharmonies

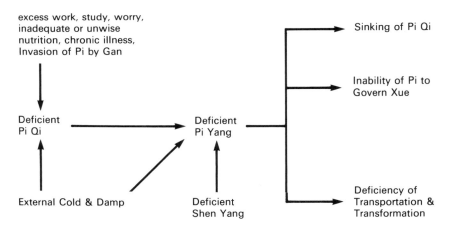

Gan

The third Zang involved in gynaecological disorders is Gan, which is linked to Deficient Shen Yin, just as Pi is linked to Deficient Shen Yang. Gan disharmonies have various origins, as shown in Figure 16.10 on page 207.

Summary

The interrelationships of Shen, Pi and Gan with the Disease Factors, in the origins of gynaecological and obstetric disorders, are shown in outline in Figure 16.11 on page 208, and discussed in greater detail elsewhere (21,22).

Figure 16.10 Origin of Gan Disharmonies

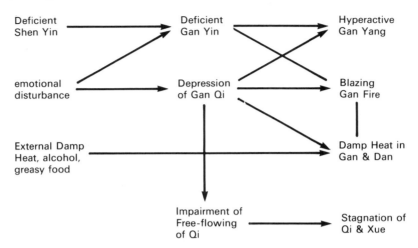

Zang Fu Interrelationships in some Common Disease Patterns

This section uses the example of some Common Disease Patterns to show the type of interrelationship of Zang Fu disharmonies and Disease Factors in the origin of disease.

Hyperthyroidism

Figure 16.12, outlining the origins of hyperthyroidism, and the Zang disharmonies and the Disease Factors involved, clearly shows the inadvisability of equating thyroid diseases with a San Jiao 'organ' (see page 62 and page 157).

Figure 16.12 Origins of Hyperthyroidism

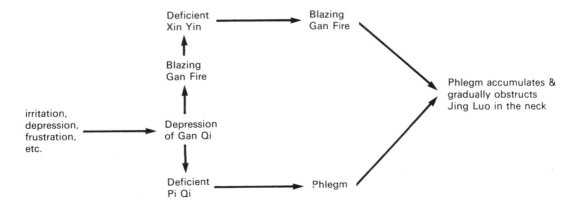

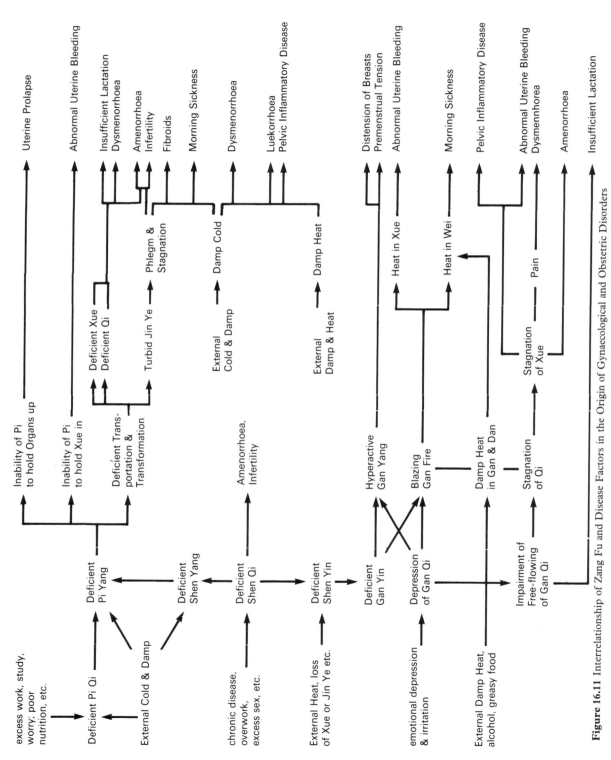

Figure 16.11 Interrelationship of Zang Fu and Disease Factors in the Origin of Gynaecological and Obstetric Disorders

Impotence

In TCM, there are three main origins of impotence:-

Excess Sex or Seminal Emission

This results in exhaustion of Shen Jing and in depletion of Ming Men and Shen Yang.

Emotional Disturbance

Fright may injure Shen Qi, and worry, anxiety, excess thinking and mental strain may injure and depress Xin and Pi.

Damp Heat Diffusing Downwards

This is a common origin of urino-genital problems, and may be associated with both External and Internal Damp. External Damp may invade the Body, or weakness of Shen and Pi may lead to accumulation of Internal Damp. Damp Heat may arise from Stagnation of Internal Damp, especially if mental irritation and frustration lead to Xin Fire which is transmitted down to Xiao Chang, or to Gan Fire which is transmitted downwards via Gan Jing Luo. Since Gan rules the Tendons, and since the Gan Tendino-muscular channel connects with the genitals, down-pouring of Damp Heat and Stagnation of Heat in Gan channel, may lead to relaxation of Muscles and Tendons, resulting in impotence.

Generally the commonest origin of impotence is Deficiency of Shen, but all the other patterns may also be involved (15).

Insomnia

There are five main origins of insomnia, which may occur singly or in combinations, depending on the predisposition of the individual, and on the prevailing situation.

Figure 16.13 Origins of Insomnia

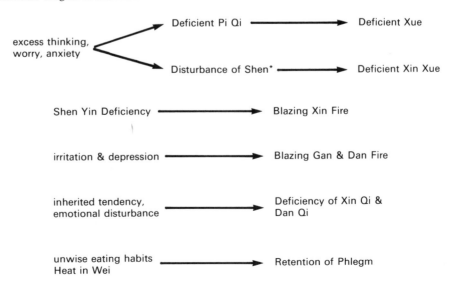

Wei Disharmonies

Wei patterns include flaccidity or atrophy of the Muscles of the limbs, with weakness or impairment of movement. Wei disharmonies involve paralysis only in the sense of flaccidity and weakness, as in polio and myasthenia, and must be distinguished from the painful disharmonies of Bi, for example arthritis and rheumatism; and from the patterns of spastic hemiparalysis of Windstroke, such as CVA sequellae and facial paralysis.

Wei patterns involve weakness and atrophy of Muscles and Tendons, due to one or more of the following:-

Figure 16.14 Origins of Wei Patterns

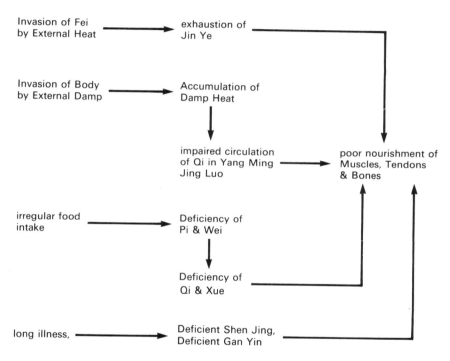

Summary

Chapter 14 considered the basis of Zang Fu interrelationships:- Yin Yang, Substances, Jing Luo and Tissues. It looked at the interrelationships between different Zang Fu, and between Zang Fu and Disease Factors in the origins of Patterns of Disharmony. Chapter 15 dealt with the interrelationship between emotional disharmony, Zang Fu disharmony, and the Origins of Disease.

This chapter investigated disharmonies involving pairs of Zang, and then combinations of three or more Zang, and progressed to four examples of Common Disease Patterns. The next stage is the study of individual case histories, to see what actually occurs in practice. To understand the methods and techniques applied in the case histories, first we must briefly consider the topics of Diagnosis, Treatment, and Patient Education, the subjects of the next chapter.

Clinical Practice

Chapter
17

Clinical Methods

The concern of this book is not with theory for its own sake, but with the application of theoretical principles in clinical practice.

The practice of Traditional Chinese acupuncture, in the People's Republic of China, is based on the clinical application of the following basic theoretical framework:-

Yin Yang   Substances
Eight Principles   Jing Luo
Disease Factors   Zang Fu

Such clinical procedures as the choice of diagnostic questions, the study of pulse and of tongue, and the choice of acupuncture points and methods of point use, are performed according to this basic framework. For example, the classification of the 28 pulse qualities is according to this theoretical framework, and any particular pulse pattern is studied in these terms. Hence a thin rapid wiry pulse may represent Deficient Yin, Deficient Heat, injury to Jin Ye, and disharmony of Gan.

However, the aim of this chapter is not to give an exhaustive description of clinical techniques, as this is given elsewhere (13,14,17,18,27), but to give an understanding of how the theoretical principles discussed in the previous chapters affect clinical practice.

The three basic areas of clinical practice are:-

Diagnosis
Treatment
Education of the Patient

Diagnosis

The first stage of clinical practice is diagnosis. Information is gathered in three main areas:-

Observation - Interrogation
Pulse
Tongue

Observation – Interrogation
It is from this method that practitioners of TCM gain most information, and it is upon this method that they most rely. It is considered to be a more important source of information than pulse or tongue. The techniques of observation - interrogation:- to see, to hear, to ask, to palpate, to smell; are familiar in the West, and will not be described here, but the concept of asking **key questions** will be emphasised.

An inexperienced practitioner may ask dozens of questions and remain confused; an experienced practitioner may cut straight to the heart of the matter with a few key questions. This is an ability that comes only with complete theoretical understanding of all the patterns of disharmony, and from many years of experience of the various permutations and combinations of these patterns in clinical practice. Three examples of the rapid resolutions provided by key questions are given below:-

1. A confusing complex of gynaecological signs was resolved by asking the question:- 'Is the pain before, during or after menstruation?' The answer that the pain was mainly before menstruation indicated that the predominant pattern would probably be Stagnation of Qi. Pain mainly during menstruation is more likely to be due to Stagnation of Xue, and pain mainly after menstruation to be associated with Deficient Qi and Deficient Xue.

2. In a case of menorrhagia it was difficult to decide whether the predominant system involved in the disharmony was Gan, Pi, Ren Mai or Chong Mai. The key question was:- 'Was there a period of heavy physical labour just before the start of the menorrhagia?' Since the lady answered that she had moved house just prior to the start of the problem, Pi was likely to be the predominant disharmony. Excess work may injure Pi, resulting in loss of the ability of Pi to Hold Xue in Xue Mai.

3. A patient complaining of sore throat with raised temperature and fast pulse was asked the question:- 'You have thirst, but do you want hot or cold drinks?' Since the answer was that the patient had no preference for hot or cold, the diagnosis was that the predominant factor was Deficient Yin. It was therefore not enough to remove the Heat from the throat, it was equally important to support the Yin. Generally, thirst with desire for cold drinks indicates Excess Heat, thirst with no preference for hot or cold drinks indicates Deficient Heat, and thirst with no desire to drink may indicate accumulation of Internal Damp. Desire for warm drinks, though not necessarily with thirst, may indicate accumulation of Cold in the Body.

Pulse

Due to inadequate information on TCM in general, and on pulse diagnosis in particular, many misconceptions and misunderstandings were incorporated into the early teaching of pulse diagnosis in Britain. Hence, the TCM pulse diagnosis that is practised in China differs greatly from that which has been taught in British schools of acupuncture in the past.

As stated above, the purpose of the methods of TCM diagnosis — observation-interrogation, pulse and tongue — is to gather information in terms of Yin Yang, Eight Principles' Patterns, Disease Factors, Substances, Jing Luo and Zang Fu.

Chinese pulse diagnosis has little concern with the Five Phases. Its purpose is to determine, for example, whether the disharmony is of Yin or Yang, of Heat or Cold, of Deficient Qi or Deficient Xue, of Pi or Gan, of Invasion by Wind Cold or Invasion by Damp, and so on.

Position and Depth

TCM pulse-taking in China is in terms of the Five Zang:- Shen, Pi, Gan, Xin and Fei; and not in terms of the Six Zang, since Xin Bao is included with Xin. Also, relatively little importance is given to the Fu systems, which are generally incorporated into their paired Zang. Hence, in contrast to the early British acupuncture pulse diagram of Table 17.1, that used in China is as in Table 17.2. In the latter figure, there is no clear separation between Zang and Fu, Xin Bao is not regarded as a separate pulse, and both right and left hand Chi positions are occupied by Shen.

Table 17.1 British Acupuncture Pulse Diagram

	Left Hand Superficial	Deep	Right Hand Deep	Superficial
Cun	Xiao Chang	Xin	Fei	Da Chang
Guan	Dan	Gan	Pi	Wei
Chi	Pang Guang	Shen	Xin Bao	San Jiao

Table 17.2 Chinese Pulse Diagram

	Left Hand		Right Hand	
Cun	(Xiao Chang)	Xin	Fei	(Da Chang)
Guan	(Dan)	Gan	Pi	(Wei)
Chi	(Pang Guang)	Shen	Shen	(San Jiao)

Western schools of acupuncture used to teach that there are two depths, superficial and deep, corresponding to Fu-and Zang respectively. There is some truth in this, in that the Fu may be considered as a Yang aspect of the Zang, but the Chinese approach to pulse-taking also includes a very different approach to depth, involving three depths:- superficial, middle and deep, which, in some applications, may be regarded as corresponding to Qi, Xue and Jing respectively.

Qualities and Quantities

The Western preoccupation was with the six pulse positions, each at two depths, giving 12 locations in total; and considerations of pulse quality were given secondary importance. The predominant Chinese concern is with the 28 pulse qualities, and with the three depths, and secondarily with the six positions corresponding to the five Zang, although these are also of importance. With the very large number of combinations of pulse qualities, at three depths and six positions, the possible permutations are enormous. This very flexible system allows classification of illness in terms of Yin Yang, Eight Principles' Patterns, Disease Factors, Substances, and Zang Fu.

Also, it was the habit in the past in the West, to describe the pulses, not in terms of qualities, but quantities. Each of the 12 Zang Fu would be marked 'plus', 'minus', or 'normal', and 'balancing' would consist in draining energy from a 'plus' to a 'minus'. The author has never seen this approach used in clinical practice in China.

Another important note is that in TCM, the pulses do **not** generally relate to **Jing Luo**; they relate to the **Zang Fu**, in terms of the Substances, Eight Principles' Patterns of Disharmony, and Disease Factors. Obviously, if a Zang is affected, its channel may also be involved, but the particular pulse pattern relates to the state of the Zang Fu and will not register changes in the channel alone.

So, in summary, the Chinese first observe the overall pulse qualities at each of the three depths, and then at each of the six positions (three on each wrist). They are looking for information in terms of Yin Yang, Eight Principles' Patterns of Disharmony, Disease Factors, Substances and Zang Fu.

Pulse Patterns of Some Common Disharmonies

Since the pulse qualities are described in detail elsewhere (12,14,27) this section concentrates on a brief outline of some of the key disharmonies (see Table 17.3).

Table 17.3 Some Basic Disharmonies with their Pulse Qualities

Disharmony	Pulse Quality	Disharmony	Pulse Quality
Deficient Yang	deep, slow	Deficiency	empty
Deficient Yin	thin, rapid	Excess	full
Deficient Qi	empty	Internal	deep
Deficient Xue	thin, choppy	External	superficial
Deficient Jing	choppy, various	Cold	slow, tight
Deficient Jin Ye	flooding	Heat	fast

Disharmony	Pulse Quality
Summer Heat	superficial, empty
Wind	superficial
Wind Heat	superficial, rapid
Wind Cold	superficial, tight
Damp	slippery
Damp Cold	slippery, slow
Damp Heat	slippery, rapid
Phlegm	slippery
Stagnant Xue	choppy, wiry
Loss of Xue	hollow

Generally, in disharmony, Shen pulse tends to be deep, since Shen rules Jing which is associated with the deep level of the pulse; Pi pulse tends to be empty, since it is often associated with Deficiency of Qi and Xue; also, since Pi and Wei form Xue, Pi is often linked with the middle depth; Gan tends to be wiry, since Gan governs smooth, even, unobstructed movement of Qi, and in disharmony tends to be associated with obstruction of Qi flow; Xin tends to be intermittent, since the regularity of the heartbeat determines the regularity of the pulse; and Fei tends to be superficial, partly because Fei deals with Qi, which is associated with the superficial level of the pulse, and partly because Fei is the uppermost Zang, the most open to Invasion by External Disease Factors. External Wind is also associated with the superficial pulse, since External Wind often represents the first stage of invasion, affecting the outermost areas of the Body.

These pulse patterns are only generalisations and, for example, a wiry pulse does not necessarily indicate Gan disharmony, nor does Summer Heat always produce a superficial and empty pulse.

Analysis of Combinations of Pulse Qualities

Pulse qualities rarely occur singly, they usually occur in combinations, indeed many qualities may be present. The art and science of pulse diagnosis is to determine clearly which qualities or combinations are present, and of these, which are predominant. The next step is to interpret these qualities, or combinations of qualities, in terms of Yin Yang, Eight Principles' Patterns, Disease Factors, Substances and Zang Fu. Few pulse patterns are unambiguous, for example the combination of slippery and rapid might indicate the presence of Damp and Heat, or it might indicate the presence of Phlegm and Fire; and a thin and choppy pulse might indicate Deficient Xue, Deficient Jing or Deficient Jin Ye; other signs would have to be considered to determine which pattern was predominant.

However, despite ambiguity, there is a clear logic in the analysis of pulse combinations. For example, some of the common combinations of the Gan disharmonies are shown in Table 17.4:-

Table 17.4 Some Common Pulse Patterns of Gan Disharmonies

Gan Disharmony	Pulse Pattern
Depression of Gan Qi	wiry
Depression of Gan Qi with Invasion of Pi & Wei, i.e. Deficiency of Pi & Wei	wiry, empty
Depression of Gan Qi with Invasion of Pi & Wei with Formation of Phlegm	wiry, slippery
Depression of Gan Qi with Stagnation of Xue	wiry, choppy
Deficient Gan Xue	wiry, thin, choppy
Deficient Gan Yin	wiry, thin, rapid
Blazing Gan Fire	wiry, full, rapid
Damp Heat in Gan & Dan	wiry, slippery, rapid
Invasion of Cold in Gan Jing Luo	wiry, slow

Obviously, there are other possible interpretations for some of these, for example, wiry and slow may indicate pain associated with Stagnation due to Cold, not necessarily associated with Gan disharmony; but these patterns form a useful general guide.

Tongue

The tongue can give information on the origins, seriousness and likely progress of a disease. Changes in the body or in the coat of the tongue can aid diagnosis and prognosis both initially and throughout the course of a treatment.

For example, a tongue that is pale, moist and slightly flabby indicates a better prognosis than a tongue that is very pale, very moist and very flabby. Also, if before treatment, the tongue were red, indicating Heat, and after treatment became normal, it would indicate treatment was successful. If, however, during treatment the tongue changed from red to scarlet, it would indicate Heat injury had become more severe, and either treatment was incorrect, or the situation had changed and required a different treatment.

The tongue is less labile than the pulse, and cannot give the same breadth and depth of information. However, like the pulse, it gives information in terms of Eight Principles' Patterns, Substances, Zang Fu and Disease Factors. Also, like the pulse, it does not give information in terms of the Jing Luo alone, but in terms of the Zang Fu. Since the study of the tongue in TCM has only been recently introduced into the West, there are fewer misconceptions regarding it, than regarding the pulse.

Tongue Patterns for some Common Disharmonies

Since study of the tongue is dealt with elsewhere (17), this section merely gives outline tongue patterns for some basic disharmonies in order to illustrate the basic theoretical framework that underlies tongue diagnosis.

Table 17.5 Some Basic Disharmonies with their Tongue Patterns

Disharmony	Tongue pattern	Disharmony	Tongue Pattern
Deficient Yang	pale, flabby, moist; ± white coat	Deficiency	thin coat
Deficient Yin	red; ± thin coat	Excess	thick coat
Deficient Qi	pale, flabby	Internal	changes in body &/or coat
Deficient Xue	pale, thin	External	changes in coat
Stagnant Xue	purple ± purple spots	Cold	pale; white coat
Deficient Jin Ye	dry, thin	Heat	red; yellow coat
Accumulation of Jin Ye	flabby, moist		

Disharmony	Tongue Pattern
Damp	moist; greasy coat
Damp Heat	red; yellow greasy coat
Phlegm	thick greasy coat
Cold Obstructing	pale purple, moist
Stagnant Xue	purple ± purple spots

These are only guidelines, for example, Deficiency is not the only origin of a thin tongue coat, which can also indicate normality, or invasion by External Disease Factors. Conversely, Deficiency might lead to Internal accumulation of food, Phlegm or Jin Ye, resulting in a thick tongue coat. Tongue patterns would never be used in isolation, only in combination with information from observation-interrogation and pulse, both of which are considered more important than data from tongue patterns.

N.B.   The tongue pattern that is sometimes described as swollen or puffy, sometimes having scalloped edges and 'toothmarks' — the apparent imprints of teeth — is termed 'flabby' in this book. This tongue pattern is usually associated with Deficient Qi, Deficient Yang, or Accumulation of Jin Ye.

Areas of the Tongue

Figure 17.1 Correspondence of Tongue Areas to Zang Fu

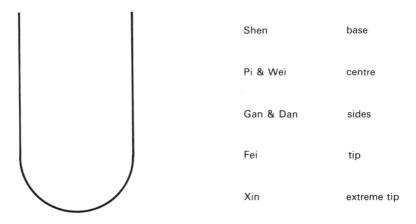

Shen	base
Pi & Wei	centre
Gan & Dan	sides
Fei	tip
Xin	extreme tip

Very roughly, the body of the tongue may be divided into areas corresponding to the Five Zang, as in Figure 17.1. However, phenomena on the centre of the tongue, for example, do not necessarily imply Pi and Wei disharmonies, any more than Pi and Wei disharmonies necessarily register only at the centre of the tongue. Nevertheless, it can be a useful guideline, for example red dots along the side of the tongue may accompany the relatively chronic Gan and Dan disharmonies, but it is necessary to remember that this may also represent acute conditions of Invasion by External Wind.

Analysis of Combinations of Tongue Characteristics
Like pulse qualities, tongue characteristics rarely occur singly, more usually in combinations. Again, Gan disharmonies are taken as an example, as in Table 17.6.
It can be seen that the information given by the tongue is less specific than that given by the pulse. There is no tongue characteristic equivalent to the wiry pulse quality, which is generally present in all Gan disharmonies, so that in some cases, the involvement of Gan in a pattern of disharmony could not be decided from the tongue alone. For example, a purple tongue merely indicates Stagnant Xue; it

would be necessary to check pulse and other clinical data to determine whether or not this Stagnant Xue were associated with Depression of Gan Qi.

Summary

The three main diagnostic techniques, in order of importance, are observation-interrogation, pulse and tongue. All three are used together to provide as clear and detailed a picture of the patient's Pattern of Disharmony as possible.

Table 17.6 Some Common Tongue Patterns of Gan Disharmonies

Gan Disharmony	Tongue Pattern
Depression of Gan Qi with Invasion of Pi by Gan	normal; white greasy coat
Depression of Gan Qi with Stagnant Xue	purple
Deficient Gan Xue	pale, ± thin & dry
eficient Gan Yin with Hyperactive Gan Yang	red, ± red dots on sides, dry; little coat
Blazing Gan Fire	red, especially sides, & perhaps tip; thick yellow dry coat
Stirring of Gan Wind	dry, ± stiff & trembling
Damp Heat in Gan & Dan	red; yellow greasy coat
Stagnation of Cold in Gan Channel	moist white coat

Differentiation of Patterns of Disharmony

Clinical practice is based on the successful differentiation of the Patterns of Disharmony involved in the patients' illness. In TCM, Disharmonies are characterised in terms of Yin Yang, Eight Principles, Disease Factors, Substances, Jing Luo and Zang Fu. The information from Observation- Interrogation, Pulse and Tongue is considered in these terms.

For example, a female patient complained of chronic restlessness and insomnia, recurring mild headaches in the temporal region, and premenstrual tension aggravated by stress and irritation. She had a wiry thin slightly rapid pulse; and tongue which was red, especially at the sides. This information was organised as follows:-

Yin Yang and Eight Principles

The condition was probably Internal, rather than External, since it was chronic and not acute. The slightly rapid pulse and red tongue with no coat indicated the condition was one of Heat rather than one of Cold. However, the mildness of the headache and the thin quality of the pulse indicated a Deficient rather than an Excess condition; and the fact that the pulse was only slightly rapid indicated it was Deficient Heat rather than Excess Heat. The combination of red tongue with no coat and thin slightly rapid pulse, indicated a Yin Deficient condition rather

220

than a Yang Deficiency. In summary, it was a chronic Internal condition of Deficient Heat, otherwise known as Deficient Yin.

Disease Factors
The red edges of the tongue could have been due to acute Invasion by Wind Heat, or they could have been associated with Disharmony of Gan and Dan. The latter was more likely, since this was a chronic condition with such signs of Gan involvement as headache and wiry pulse. The precipitating factor may have been predominantly emotional, since the premenstrual tension was aggravated by stress and irritation. In summary, the Disease Factors may have been predominantly Internal, associated with emotional disharmony.

Substances
Some Deficiency of Jin Ye may have been involved in the Yin Deficiency condition, since there were signs of both Deficiency and of Heat, for example thin, rapid pulse and red tongue. Also, some Disturbance of Shen* may have been involved in the insomnia and restlessness, associated with Blazing Gan Fire affecting Xin. In summary, Deficiency of Jin Ye and Disturbance of Shen* were the two most likely Patterns of Disharmony of the Substances here.

Jing Luo and Zang Fu
The first question was whether this illness involved Jing Luo only, or whether Zang Fu were also involved. Since pathological changes were registered on pulse and tongue, Zang Fu must have been involved here. This idea was reinforced by the presence of such chronic Internal signs as changes in the menstrual cycle. That the Dan channel was involved was shown by the location of the headache, but this was predominantly a Zang Fu rather than a Jing Luo pattern.

The second question was concerned with which Zang Fu were involved. The wiry pulse suggested Gan and perhaps Dan, the headache suggested Gan and/or Dan, and the temporal location of the headache suggested Dan.

The third question was which Pattern of Disharmony of Gan and Dan was involved. The premenstrual tension suggested Hyperactive Gan Yang, as did the headache; and the thin slightly rapid pulse, and red tongue with little coat suggested the Hyperactive Gan Yang was associated with Deficient Gan Yin.

In summary, in this Pattern of Disharmony, Zang Fu predominated, rather than Jing Luo; specifically it was Deficient Yin and Hyperactive Yang of Gan, with involvement of Dan Jing Luo.

This woman's illness could therefore be described as a condition of Deficient Internal Heat, originating from emotional disharmony, involving Deficiency of Jin Ye and Disturbance of Shen*, and termed Deficient Yin and Hyperactive Yang of Gan, with involvement of Dan Jing Luo.

Treatment

Having gathered information from observation-interrogation, pulse and tongue, and on the basis of this data having correctly differentiated the Patterns of Disharmony involved, the next stage is treatment. Proper treatment involves the correct selection, location and use of acupuncture points for the particular Pattern of Disharmony.

Choice of Points

As seen in Chapter 5, each of the Common Disease Patterns is organised in terms of Yin Yang, Eight Principles' Patterns, Disease Factors, Substances, Jing Luo and Zang Fu, and for every patient the points used are selected according to these principles. For example, in cases of premenstrual tension and headache, of the type given in the example above:-

Yin Yang and Eight Principles' Patterns

For Internal Deficient Heat, i.e. Deficient Yin, points would be used to nourish the Yin, for example, Sanyinjiao, SP.6, and Taixi, KID.3.

Disease Factors

For Internal emotional disharmony of the type related to restlessness and insomnia, points such as Yinxi, HE.6, Shenmen, HE.7, Yintang, M-HN-3,and Anmian, M-HN-54, could be used to pacify Xin and mind. For emotional disharmony of the type related to irritation and premenstrual tension, Taichong, LIV.3, could be used to pacify Gan.

Substances

For Disturbance of Shen*, the points listed for restlessness and insomnia could be used, and for Deficiency of Jin Ye, the points listed for Deficient Yin could be applied.

Zang Fu and Jing Luo

For the pattern of Deficient Gan Yin, points such as Sanyinjiao and Taixi could be used, and for the Hyperactive Gan Yang, with invasion of Dan channel, points such as Taichong, Fengchi, GB.20, and Baihui, Du 20; could be used to pacify Gan and to regulate the Hyperactive Yang in the head.

In summary, in such cases, points such as Taichong, Fengchi, Baihui, Sanyinjiao, Taixi, Yinxi, Shenmen, Yintang and Anmian, could be used for the reasons stated. *But* this is only a theoretical example, and actual patients would be assessed according to their individual needs, at the time of treatment.

Use of Points

Following correct selection and location of the acupuncture points, the next step is correct point use. In this, there are three main aspects:-

Correct Choice of Method of Use
Production of Needle Sensation
Correct Technique of Insertion - Manipulation

Correct Choice of Method of Point Use

The main method is acupuncture needle with manual manipulation, but there are many other techniques; for example, moxibustion, cupping, bleeding, tapping, embedding, electro-acupuncture, and so on. Since these techniques are dealt with in detail elsewhere (13), they will not be discussed here.

222

Production of Needle Sensation

With good needle insertion technique, the patient may or may not experience a pin-prick as the needle pierces the skin; but if the needle is blunt, or inserted too slowly, piercing the skin may be distinctly painful. However, once the needle is through the skin, the practitioner aims to produce a quite separate feeling:- De Qi or 'the needle sensation'. This is felt as a sensation of numbness, soreness, heaviness, aching or distension; and some patients may feel a sensation of heat or cold, or a sensation like a dull electric shock. This sensation is distinct from the pain which may follow if there is incorrect location of the point, or if the needle grates against bone, pierces a blood vessel, penetrates a main nerve, or becomes entangled in a tendon. It is important that both practitioner and patient can distinguish between pain and the true needle sensation. The latter may be uncomfortable, but it is distinct from pain. De Qi indicates correct location of the point and pain indicates incorrect location, except for some points, such as those on the palms and soles, and on the tips of the fingers and toes, which are definitely painful, even on correct location. Also, although De Qi is usually obtained from points on limbs and body, practitioners may not attempt to produce sensations of soreness etc, on head and face; some merely insert and gently manipulate, avoiding any strong sensation, others aim to produce mild feelings of distension only.

De Qi, 'needle sensation', or 'needle reaction', is said to indicate the 'arrival of Qi' at the acupuncture point. The importance of 'obtaining Qi' cannot be over-emphasised, and if it is not obtained after insertion, various methods of needle manipulation should be used until it arrives. However, in weak patients, De Qi may be difficult to obtain, it may only come slowly or perhaps not at all. Generally, if De Qi comes quickly and easily, it is a good prognosis, indicating the patient has sufficient Qi within the channels to assist recovery. If De Qi is hard to obtain, it may indicate a poor prognosis, and a slow recovery. However, De Qi may come more easily as treatment progresses, and the strength of the patient increases. For some acupuncture points, and for some patients, De Qi may always be poor, although treatment brings results; but as a general rule, presence of De Qi indicates the correct location of a point, and the likelihood of a good response to treatment, and absence of De Qi indicates incorrect location or the likelihood of a poor response.

Correct Technique of Insertion - Manipulation

The topic is dealt with in detail elsewhere (13,18), and indeed the variety of different techniques is often confusing to the student. Whilst the more complex techniques, with their lovely names like 'Battle of the Tiger and Dragon', and the 'Male and Female Phoenix Ruffle their Wings', may have validity in certain situations, it is important that the student understands the basic principles of manipulation technique, before moving on to the complexities.

The three fundamental methods of needle manipulation are related to the three basic conditions of disharmony:-

Excess
Deficiency
Intermediate or Mixed

Excess conditions must be reduced, Deficient conditions must be reinforced, and Intermediate conditions balanced. In Table 17.7, the three main methods of needle manipulation are listed, along with the associated conditions for which they are used, the type of manipulation adopted by the practitioner, and the type of sensation felt by the patient:-

Table 17.7 The Three Basic Methods of Needle Manipulation

Method	Condition	Manipulation	Sensation
Reinforcing	Deficiency	gentle, slow, small	gentle
Even	Intermediate or Mixed	moderate	moderate
Reducing	Excess	strong, fast, large	strong

Whether reinforcing, even or reducing method is used, the needle is inserted and De Qi obtained in every case. The difference between the three methods lies in the **strength** of the needle sensation felt by the patient, and in the **type of manipulation** used by the practitioner to obtain it.

In the case of Deficiency, especially in a patient with a weak constitution, gentle manipulation is used, so that the needle sensation is gentle, in order to reinforce gently and to strengthen the Deficiency. If strong manipulation is used, producing strong needle sensation, the patient may simply faint, because his energy is weak, and, in the West, be reluctant to return for treatment. On the other hand, if the patient is suffering from an Excess condition, for example, severe pain or fever, gentle needle sensation may not be sufficient to reduce the Excess. Nevertheless, although strong manipulation is especially appropriate for a condition of Excess in a patient with strong constitution, in an Excess condition in a patient with a weak constitution, it is best to observe caution, and not to use excessively strong manipulation, or again the patient may lose consciousness.

Severe pain is generally associated with an Excess condition, and the analgesic effect of electro-acupuncture in such cases is seen as reducing method, equivalent to strong manual manipulation of the needles. For example, medical and dental operations, childbirth, and conditions of extreme pain in general practice, such as trigeminal neuralgia. In Asia, fevers are a common category of Excess condition in the form of acute Internal Heat. The heat is reduced by the use of appropriate points using reducing method, using strong stimulation without retaining the needles, or, alternatively, retaining the needles and manipulating intermittently. For example, malaria or bacterial dysentery. Such febrile diseases are rarely treated by acupuncture in the West, where the majority of cases met with in general practice are those of Deficiency and/or Stagnation. Whilst reducing method may be used to remove local stagnation in the channel and area, for example the use of Tiakou, ST.38, for frozen shoulder, or Neihegu, N-UE-17, for neck sprain, in the West, reinforcing and even method are more commonly used than reducing method.

Generally, acute conditions have aspects of Excess, even if they are based on underlying Deficiency. In such cases, reducing method might be used during the acute Excess phase, and reinforcing method might be used between acute attacks to strengthen the underlying Deficiency. However, even in the acute phase, it may be safer to use even method, if the patient is especially weak, or fainting may occur.

Summary

Successful treatment relies on the correct selection of the points, their accurate location, and, if manual insertion of acupuncture needle is the appropriate general method, on the proper use of the appropriate type of needle manipulation. Also, it is generally essential to obtain De Qi.

There are three basic conditions:- Excess, Deficiency and Intermediate. To reduce Excess conditions, the practitioner uses strong manipulation, so that the patient feels a strong needle sensation. To reinforce Deficiency, gentle manipulation is used to produce a gentle needle sensation. In conditions that are intermediate between Excess and Deficiency, or in conditions that contain aspects of both Excess and Deficiency, the even method is used, with moderate manipulation and needle sensation.

Education of the Patient

The aim of diagnosis is the clear perception of the different Patterns of Disharmony involved in the patient's illness. This enables correct choice of points and method of point use. Also, once the different originating and aggravating factors of the illness are understood by the practitioner, this understanding can be transmitted to the patient, so that he or she can take the necessary steps to avoid or to reduce these factors. Treatment and education combine to relieve the disharmony, and the practitioner and patient work together to remedy the disease. In some simple situations, treatment alone may be sufficient, in others the disharmony may be redressed solely by the remedial actions of the patient. Generally, however, both the acupuncture treatment and the correct remedial measures carried out by the patient are required to achieve lasting improvement. This is especially true in the complex cases of chronic Deficiency seen in the West. Unless the patient is given a clear understanding of the origins of the illness, and shown what remedial procedures to adopt, the disharmony may drag on indefinitely, although partly relieved by acupuncture treatment. In other words, the appropriate actions of patients to help themselves can greatly reduce their sufferings and their need for acupuncture or other medical treatment.

There are two main aspects of patient education. The first is concerned with the identification of the originating factors of the illness, and then with prescribing the appropriate remedial measures to these factors and to the pathological changes associated with them. The second is concerned with helping patients at a more personal level. To help people to help themselves it is first necessary to help them to understand themselves, then to accept themselves, and yet also to determine to change themselves. This is the basis of patient education.

Identification of Originating Factors and Selection of Appropriate Remedial Measures

This section relates back to the chapter on Origins of Disease, since the aim of patient education is to identify the originating factors, and then to show the patient how to avoid or reduce them. The three main categories of originating factors are External, Internal, and Neither Internal nor External. The three tables below list each originating factor with an example of appropriate preventative or remedial measure, and give an example of a Common Disease Pattern in which the originating factor may be involved.

Some of these preventative and remedial measures may seem absurdly obvious, yet, if people consistently adopted these measures, there would be little ill- health and disease left in this world. People are either ignorant of them, or unwisely

Table 17.8 External Factors - Climate

Factor	Remedy	Disharmony
Wind	avoid exposure to wind	common cold
Cold	avoid exposure to cold	acute asthma
Heat	avoid exposure of skin to Wind & Heat	some cases of acute urticaria
Damp	avoid damp surroundings, damp clothes etc.	fixed Bi
Dryness	avoid dry atmospheres	dry cough
Summer Heat	avoid excess exposure to sun	sunstroke

Table 17.9 Internal Factors - Emotions

Factor	Remedy	Disharmony
Joy	breathing, relaxation & meditation exercises; moderation of social life etc.	insomnia
Anger	as for Joy; physical exercise; avoid alcohol & rich, greasy food, etc.	headache
Grief, Sadness	increased & more varied social life, helping others, etc.	cardiac insufficiency
Pensiveness	iron supplement; reduce source of worry; reduce study & excess thinking; increase out-going & relaxing activity	anaemia
Fear, Fright	avoid Cold, especially in lumbar area rest & relaxation; avoid sources of fright; etc.	urinary incontinence

Table 17.10 Miscellaneous Factors

Factor	Remedy	Disharmony
Nutrition	regularize eating habits, balance diet, avoid excess greasy foods; etc.	epigastric pain
Overwork	reduce workload; correct posture & usage; avoid Cold & lifting; etc.	chronic lumbar pain
Occupational	correct stooped posture; improve breathing; outdoor exercise; avoid excessive Cold; etc.	chronic bronchitis
Deficient Exercise	vigorous exercise of whole body, specific abdominal exercises; avoid excess Cold & exertion at period times, etc.	irregular menstruation
Relationships	counselling, both of individual & couple; relaxation, breathing & meditation exercises etc.	impotence
Sex	reduce sexual activity; reduce excess mental & physical work; avoid unnecessary stress; etc.	haematuria
Trauma	increase & regularize sleep; reduce drugs; reduce workload; avoid stress; etc.	proneness to accidents

ignore them for various reasons. Patient education therefore consists in giving patients a clear picture of the originating factors of their illness, and in showing them the appropriate measures of self-help.

We will now consider some of the examples listed in the tables in a little more detail.

Common Cold

Invasion of Fei by External Wind Cold may result in impairment of the Dispersing function of Fei, just as the latter may facilitate Invasion by Wind Cold. This Wind Cold may give rise to Heat in Fei, due to the Stagnation resulting from the weak Dispersing function, and, in turn, this Heat may weaken the Dispersing function further. The Deficiency of the Dispersing function of Fei, and Heat in Fei, are both aggravated by the habit of smoking.

If Pi Qi is Deficient, and insufficient Gu Qi is formed, then Fei Qi may become Deficient, and the Dispersing function of Fei may be reduced. Also, if the weakness of Pi Qi leads to the formation of Phlegm, this may accumulate in Fei, due to the retardation of the Dispersing function, which it further weakens.

Figure 17.2 Origins of the Common Cold

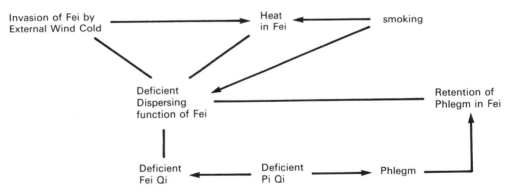

Remedial measures might include:-
1. Avoid External Disease Factors such as Wind and Cold.
2. Breathing exercises and physical exercises to strengthen Fei Qi and the Dispersing function of Fei, to disperse Phlegm.
3. Stop smoking to reduce Heat in Fei, and to avoid further damage to Fei Qi.
4. Improve diet and regularize eating habits to increase Pi Qi, and hence Fei Qi and Defensive Qi, and hence to increase the resistance of the Body to External Invasion.

Headache

Headache may be associated with many Disease Factors and with many Patterns of Disharmony. It may arise from Invasion by Wind Cold, Wind Heat or Wind Damp; from Deficient Shen Yin or Deficient Shen Yang. It may be associated with Deficient Xue, Deficient Pi Qi, or Turbid Mucus in the upper Body; it may result from trauma and from Stagnant Xue. Especially, it often occurs with Patterns of

Disharmonies of Gan and Dan, especially Depression of Gan Qi, Hyperactive Gan Yang, Blazing Gan Fire and Stirring of Gan Wind.

Assume a situation where anger and frustration are associated with Depression of Gan Qi, and with uprising of Gan Yang. Mental irritation is associated with Deficient Shen Yin and Deficient Gan Yin, again giving rise to Hyperactive Gan Yang. This results in disturbance of movement of Qi in the channels of the head, especially in channels of Gan and Dan, which is further aggravated by the Invasion of the head and neck by External Wind Cold.

In such a case, the patient could take the following measures to avoid or to reduce the force of the precipitating factors:-

1. Avoid exposure of head and neck to Wind Cold.
2. Avoid situations of stress and emotional flare-up.
3. Avoid irregular patterns generally, and especially those of irregular and insufficient sleep, to avoid aggravation of Deficient Shen Yin, and hence Deficient Gan Yin.
4. Avoid alcohol and greasy food which might aggravate the flaring of Depression of Gan Qi into Hyperactive Yang or Blazing Fire.

Haematuria
Haematuria, the occurrence of blood in the urine, may result from one or more of the following factors:-

Trauma
Physical injury to a part of the urinary system: kidneys, ureters, bladder or urethra.

Physical Overwork
This can weaken Shen Qi, so that Shen Qi descends; and Pi Qi, so that Pi cannot properly hold Xue in Xue Mai; resulting in haematuria.

Chronic Illness
This can also weaken Qi of Shen and Pi, resulting in blood in the urine.

Excess Sex
Depending on the inherent tendency of the patient, and upon the circumstances, excess sex can weaken either Shen Yin or Shen Yang. Deficient Shen Yin may give rise to Heat within Shen, which may result in bleeding directly, or via Gan or Xin Fire. Deficient Shen Yang may give rise to Deficient Pi Yang, and the two together may result in the inability of Yang Qi to hold Xue in Xue Mai, as with chronic illness and physical overwork.

Emotional Disturbance
Fear and fright may give rise to weakness of Shen Qi, but the commoner emotional origins of haematuria are stress, mental irritation, mental overwork, and frustration and anger, giving rise to Deficient Shen Yin, Blazing Gan Fire, and Blazing Xin Fire. If Xin Fire is transmitted downwards via Xiao Chang, it may reach Pang Guang, causing inflammation, irritation and haematuria. Also, Gan Fire may be

transmitted downwards via Gan Jing Luo which connects with the uro-genital area, to Pang Guang, with similar results. The Heat accumulating in Pang Guang from one or more of these sources, may result in Heat in Xue, and in subsequent leakage of Xue from Xue Mai.

Hence, appropriate remedial measures for the patient might include:-

1. Avoidance of excess physical work or exercise, whilst the injury heals, and whilst Shen and Pi Qi regain strength. Avoidance of External Cold and Damp.
2. Avoidance of excess sex, especially when emotionally upset, tired, ill, or whilst recuperating from chronic or acute illness.
3. Avoidance of mental overwork, mental stress and emotional upset. Regular and adequate rhythm of nutrition, rest and sleep, to nourish Yin, so that it may control Fire.

The common cold was taken from the table of External Factors, headache from the table of Internal Factors, and Haematuria from the table of Miscellaneous Factors. However, in clinical practice, as can be seen from these three examples, Disease Factors of all three types may be involved in a single disharmony.

Helping Patients to Help Themselves

In the West, the main origins of disease are not physical factors, but disharmonious patterns of thought and emotion (20). Changing these ingrained Patterns of Disharmony is the most important, but the most difficult, part of patient education, since most people are distinctly reluctant to change their personalities. The regulation of these deeply embedded patterns of feeling and belief is the core of patient education. Since some individuals cannot cope with this at all, and since most people can only deal with change in limited amounts, progress must be gradual, a little at a time, and only at a rate within the capacity of the patient. There are three components to the basic formula for change:-

Understanding
Motivation
Discipline

Understanding

Patients must first understand, as thoroughly as is appropriate, the pattern of their disharmony in the context of the pattern of their lives. They need to know which aspects of their make-up or behaviour became the originating factors of their illness. In this way they can understand which of their patterns of thought, emotion and behaviour need to be modified, and thus which preventative and remedial measures are appropriate.

Motivation

Understanding alone is not enough. There must be the motivation to put the understanding into practice. This can only come from within the patient; the practitioner may act as a catalyst, but cannot supply motivation to a person who altogether lacks it.

Discipline

Momentary enthusiasm, temporary motivation, is useless. Changing ingrained patterns of thought and emotion is the work of a lifetime. Discipline is the steady application of understanding and motivation over long periods of time, despite setbacks and discouragements. This is the only way that lasting change can be effective. Discipline does **not** mean sudden, harsh bursts of self torture and deprivation; it is the slow, steady, gentle implementation of change, discarding the deleterious, and nurturing the useful.

Summary

The education of the patient rests on the foundation of the clear perception by the practitioner of the patient's disorder in the context of the patient's life and environment. The practitioner must then communicate this understanding to the patient. From this understanding and from the practitioner's encouragement and support, the desire and motivation for change may arise within the patient. If the patient can develop the discipline to sustain this motivation and to apply the understanding over a period of time, he has the means for long-term health.

More specifically, the practitioner needs to know the appropriate remedial measures for different disharmonies and different situations, and the patient, once informed of them, needs to carry them out.

Summary of the Sequence of Clinical Procedures

Let us assume that a patient comes to the surgery complaining of ache and soreness in the lumber region. What would be the likely sequence of clinical procedures, and what is the logic behind them?

Preliminaries

It is assumed that the practitioner is physically fit and mentally calm. The practitioner must be completely fluent with all the theoretical principles, and be familiar with all the main Patterns of Disharmony and Common Disease Patterns and their common permutations and combinations in clinical practice. The practitioner must also be competent with all the major techniques of diagnosis and treatment, and be perceptive and supportive in dealing with the patient.

The Sequence

As soon as the patient walks through the door of the surgery, the practitioner is starting to build up an understanding of the patient's Pattern of Disharmony. The practitioner seeks to organise information from the three main areas of diagnosis — observation-interrogation, pulse and tongue — in terms of the basic framework of TCM:- Yin Yang, Eight Principles, Disease Factors, and the Patterns of Disharmony of Substances, Jing Luo and Zang Fu.

General Principles

Acute or Chronic

The first question concerns whether the disease is acute or chronic. If acute, is it genuinely acute or is this an acute crisis on an underlying chronic pattern?

Eight Principles' Patterns of Disharmony
The next questions involve the Eight Principles' Patterns of Disharmony. Is the disease External or Internal; and if External, is it purely External, or External due to, or mixed with, an underlying Internal pattern? Is it a pattern of Heat or Cold, an oscillation between, or a combination of both Heat and Cold? Is it a pattern of Excess or Deficiency, and if Excess, is it a genuine Excess, or is it temporary or a local Excess, on an underlying pattern of Deficiency? Finally, is it a Yin pattern or a Yang pattern?

Disease Factors
It is also necessary to know which Disease Factors are involved; External Factors such as Wind and Cold, Internal Factors such as anger and fear, Miscellaneous Factors such as trauma and malnutrition, may all be involved.

Substances, Jing Luo and Zang Fu
The practitioner aims to determine which Patterns of Disharmony of the Substances are involved, such as Deficient Qi or Stagnant Xue; whether this is a disharmony predominantly of Jing Luo or Zang Fu; and which Jing Luo or Zang Fu are involved.

Backache in General

Acute or Chronic
The backache may be purely acute, due to recent trauma, with resulting local Stagnation of Qi and Xue. Alternatively, an accident of years ago might have left an area of potential weakness of circulation of Qi and Xue, that is periodically activated by Invasion of Wind Cold.

Eight Principles' Patterns of Disharmony
Exposure to extreme Wind, Cold and Damp, may give rise to an acute External condition; congenital weakness of the lumbar area may be associated with a chronic Internal pattern; or the latter may predispose to Invasion by External Disease Factors, producing a chronic Internal condition with periodic acute crises due to External Invasion.

   The condition may be associated with Cold or with Heat, whether External or Internal. Alternatively, Internal Cold and Damp in the Body may give rise to Damp Heat, and finally the pain may be associated with either Deficient Yin or Deficient Yang.

Disease Factors
The main External Disease Factors involved include Wind, Cold and Damp. The main Internal Disease Factors involved include fear and fright that may injure Shen Qi and Shen Yang, and mental and emotional stress that may injure Shen Yin. The main miscellaneous Disease Factors involved are insufficient, excess or inappropriate exercise; overwork, excess sex, inherited tendency, trauma, malnutrition and occupation or general poor posture and usage.

Substances, Jing Luo and Zang Fu
The common Substance disharmonies in lumbar conditions are Deficient Qi, Deficient Jing, and Stagnant Qi and Xue. This may be in terms of Jing Luo alone, specifically those of Pang Guang and Du Mai; or, in addition, Zang Fu may be involved, specifically Shen, for example Deficient Shen Qi, Deficient Shen Jing, Deficient Shen Yin or Deficient Shen Yang. Alternatively, the downward pouring of Damp Heat into Pang Guang, discussed on page 80, may include among its signs stabbing or severe lumbar pain that is associated with urinary stones, dysuria or haematuria. In female patients, lumbar pain may be associated with menstrual disorders or with pregnancy.

A Specific Case of Lumbar Pain
Clinical situations are rarely simple; there is rarely a single originating factor, but usually a combination of various factors. Let us take a specific case.

A man of 30 years of age came from a family prone to lumbar pain. At the ages of 18 and 20, he had accidents involving the lower back, but no subsequent problems at that time. From 22, he started his own business which involved much overwork, tiredness and stress. At 24, in an attempt to regain physical fitness, he started weight-lifting. From 23 onwards, he had more or less continual lumbar soreness, worse in winter, and generally aggravated by Cold and Damp. At 30, in addition to this, he had a stabbing pain in his left lumbo-sacral area, following a session of weight-lifting, and persisting until the patient first came for treatment.

The practitioner perceived the pattern as follows. It was a chronic condition with periodic crises occurring for various reasons. There was an underlying potential weakness in the circulation of Qi and Xue in this area, due to both inherited tendency and early trauma. This pattern of weakness manifested as lumbar pain, when the weakness was aggravated by overwork, tiredness and stress. These factors injured Shen Qi, Shen Yang, and Shen Yin, increasing the weakness of circulation of Qi and Xue in the lumbar area. This disharmony was therefore not solely one of Jing Luo, but of both Jing Luo and Zang Fu. Since excess work or lifting injures Shen, this condition was exacerbated by the weight-lifting, which, in itself, and in moderation, is a useful exercise, but unwise in this case. The patterns of Deficient Qi and Stagnant Qi and Xue in the channels and collaterals of the lumbar area were worsened by the Invasion of External Cold and Damp, factors tending to retard and obstruct the flow of Qi. Also, prolonged exposure to Cold and Damp tends to injure Shen Yang. Finally, the weakened state of the back resulted in a local injury during weight-lifting, associated in TCM with Stagnant Xue.

In this case, the Principle of Treatment was to warm and strengthen Shen Qi and Shen Yang, in order to strengthen the circulation of Qi and Xue in the lumbar region, and to disperse the accumulation of Cold and Damp. Points selected in this context were used with reinforcing method and moxa. In addition, points were used with even method and moxa to relieve pain and disperse Stagnation in the area of the recent injury.

| Shenshu | BL.23 | To strengthen Shen Qi and disperse Cold and Damp. |
| Mingmen | Du 4 | To strengthen Shen Yang and to strengthen back. |

232

Weizhong	BL.54	Added since there was a history of Stagnation of Qi and Xue, and also because there was a recent acute pain below the level of Shenshu. (If the blood vessels in the popliteal fossa appear congested it is permissible to use strong stimulation or to prick Weizhong to produce a drop of blood.)
Kunlun	BL.60	As a point for chronic lumbar pain, to remove obstruction from the collaterals of the back.
Guanyuanshu	BL.26	Added, on the left side only, to relieve pain and Stagnation following the recent injury.

The patient was given a clear understanding of the origin of his back problem, and its likely future progression. He was advised to avoid exposure to Cold and Damp, to stop weight-lifting, at least temporarily, and to put more emphasis on swimming and on other relatively gentle exercises, to keep the back both invigorated and supple. He was advised to attempt to reduce overwork, with its attendant stress and tiredness, and to get more sleep and rest, to rebuild Shen Qi. The importance of regular eating habits and of adequate nutrition was emphasised, since the replaceable part of Shen Jing derives from food and drink and the action of Pi Qi.

Summary

The three main areas of clinical practice are diagnosis, treatment and patient education.

The three main methods of gaining information in diagnosis are observation-interrogation, pulse and tongue.

In differential diagnosis, this information is organized in terms of Yin Yang, Eight Principles, Disease Factors, Substances, Jing Luo and Zang Fu; and choice of principles of treatment, of points, of methods of point use, and of modes of patient education, are decided on this basis. A simple sequence of clinical procedures was outlined, using the example of lumbar pain.

Chapter
18

Case Histories

The previous chapter discussed the principles of clinical practice. Outlines of eight case histories are given below to illustrate the application of these principles in the surgery, with actual individual patients.

1. Chronic Otitis Media

A woman of 23 had had otitis media for 10 years, during which time the disease had waxed and waned. A recent attack had started 6 days before coming for treatment, and involved pain and watery discharge in the left ear, with impaired hearing and dizziness. Her pulse was slightly wiry and slightly rapid, and her tongue was red with a moist thin coat.

Diagnosis
There are two main types of otitis media:- Excess and Deficient. The Excess type is mainly associated with Damp Heat in Gan and Dan, which goes upward to disturb the ear. Signs are severe burning pain in the ear, referring to the head; and when the eardrum is perforated, there may be sticky yellow pus, and perhaps fever. The pulse is rapid and wiry, and the tongue coat is yellow. This is the acute otitis of Western medicine.

The Deficient type is mainly associated with Deficiency of Shen and Gan, with hyperactive Fire ascending to disturb the ear. Discharge is thinner and more watery than with Excess type. In repeated attacks there may be dizziness, tinnitus, and impaired hearing, associated with Shen Deficiency. Pulse is thin and wiry, and tongue red with a thin yellowish coat.

This patient showed an acute exacerbation of chronic otitis of the Deficient type.

Treatment

The principle of Treatment was to strengthen the Body, especially Shen and Gan, to disperse Fire and ease the ear.

The points used were:-

Zusanli	ST.36	Strengthens Body and its resistance to infection and inflammation.
Qiuxu	GB.40 ⎱	Soothe Gan and Dan, and regulate ear, since Dan
Tinghui	GB. 2 ⎰	channel passes through it.
Yifeng	TB.17	Local point of San Jiao channel, which passes through the ear; strengthens effect of soothing Fire of Gan and Dan.
Taixi	KID.3	Strengthens Shen to relieve Damp, and strengthens Shen Yin to eliminate Heat. Strengthens Jing Qi to aid ear.

Since this case was of underlying Deficiency, needles were used with Reinforcing method, with gentle lifting and thrusting and rotation manipulation. Needles were retained for 20 minutes, and the ear points were inserted to a depth of about half an inch only.

After one treatment, the watery discharge ceased, and the pain in the ear subsided. Two more treatments were given using the same points, and then the patient was sent to the Ear, Nose and Throat department for examination. Only a slight congestion of the tympanic membrane was observed to remain. Two more treatments were given to consolidate the healing, and the patient was discharged.

Patient Education

The patient was advised to avoid exposure to Cold, and not to allow water in the ear.

2. Tinnitus and Balance

A man of 50, under stress for many years, lost his mother and brother in close succession. He began to feel very ill, with severe dizziness and nausea, and was taken to hospital, where his speech became garbled and he became paralysed down the left side. The speech defect and paralysis disappeared in approximately 2 weeks, leaving him with vertigo, tinnitus and a sensation of discomfort in the neck. He had had catarrh for many years; had a wiry slippery pulse; and a tongue with a thick greasy coat. His condition was aggravated by exposure to Wind and Cold.

Diagnosis

Stress and bereavement resulted in Depression of Gan Qi, Hyperactivity of Gan Yang, and Stirring of Gan Wind, which, combined with the upward movement of Phlegm, led to Windstroke; with dizziness, temporary paralysis and difficulty of speech, and wiry pulse. The presence of Phlegm resulted in catarrh, nausea, slippery pulse, and thick greasy tongue coat. Deficiency of Shen Qi was involved in the tinnitus; and Deficient Shen Yin, and hence Deficient Gan Yin, were involved in the Hyperactivity of Gan Yang. External Wind and Cold aggravated the condition by further disturbance and obstruction of the circulation of Qi and Xue in the channels and collaterals of the head.

Treatment
The principle of treatment was to pacify Hyperactive Gan Yang, resolve Phlegm, strengthen Shen, and to disperse External Wind and Cold and clear the channels of the head and ears. Points were selected from such as the following, and used with even method.

Fengchi, Yifeng and Yiming were used with moxa in addition to needle, and after this was done, the patient covered these points with a scarf until he got home, to avoid a sudden fall in temperature at these points, i.e. exposure to Wind Cold.

Zulinqi	GB.41 ⎱	Confluent points of Tai Mai and Yang Wei Mai.
Waiguan	TB.5 ⎰	In combination with other Dan and San Jiao points, used to clear obstruction from these Jing Luo. Waiguan also clears External problems, for example Wind and Cold.
Fengchi	GB.20	Pacifies Hyperactive Gan Yang and Internal Wind. Also clears External conditions, in this case Wind and Cold.
Ermen	TB.21 ⎱	Clear channels of the ear and dispel Wind.
Yifeng	TB.17 ⎰	
Yiming	M-HN-13	Specific for vertigo and tinnitus.
Baihui	Du 20	Calms turbulent Yang in the head.
Taichong	LIV.3	Calms Hyperactive Gan Yang.
Yongquan	KID.1	Strengthens Yin and calms Hyperactive Yang.
Taixi	KID.3	Strengthens Shen Qi and Shen Yin.
Fenglong	ST.40 ⎱	
Zusanli	ST.36 ⎬	Strengthen Pi and Wei to transform Phlegm.
Zhongwan	Ren 12 ⎰	

Patient Education
There were two main aspects:- reduction of Phlegm, and reduction of tension. The patient was advised to avoid chronic build-up of tension in various ways, and he co-operated fully in this. In order to reduce Phlegm, he reduced his smoking habit, had periodic cleansing diets, and adjusted his general diet to avoid Phlegm-forming foods.

In addition, he was advised to avoid overwork, so that Shen Qi might slowly rebuild, and to avoid exposure of his head and neck to Wind and Cold.

The tinnitus was almost completely removed after four treatments, and subsequently both tinnitus and vertigo have been maintained at minimal levels by regular treatment, once every 1 or 2 months.

3.   Angina Pectoris

For six years, a man of 50 had chest pain and breathlessness only on exertion. For a period of 4 days, 1 year ago, he had continual chest pain, which was then diagnosed as a mild heart attack. Members of his family also had had heart conditions, and he had suffered from nervousness and insomnia since he was a boy. He had been involved in several serious car accidents, and for many years had severe stress in his business and was a great worrier. The bouts of chest pain were initiated or aggravated by exertion, cold or stress. He had palpitations, felt the cold, had difficulty in urinating; had a wiry slightly slow pulse; and a pale flabby tongue.

Diagnosis

The chest pain, palpitations, nervousness and insomnia indicated a Xin disorder. Since pain was the dominant factor, Stagnation of Xin Xue was the main disharmony, although cyanosis was only slight in this case, and the tongue was pale rather than purple. The pale tongue indicated Deficient Yang, Deficient Qi and Deficient Xue. The sensitivity to Cold, aggravation of chest pain by Cold, slightly slow pulse and flabby tongue indicated Deficient Yang. Deficiency of Qi and Yang of Shen, led to the inability of Shen to hold down Qi sent by Fei, leading to breathlessness on exertion. It also led to impairment of Jin Ye metabolism, involving difficult urination.

In addition to the inherent tendency to Xin weakness, various emotional stresses contributed to this condition. Firstly, the Shen-Xin relationship had been weakened by the severe fear, fright and shock involved in the series of car accidents. This resulted in Deficient Qi and Yang of Shen and Xin. Secondly, the Pi-Xin relationship may have been weakened by the continual chronic worry, resulting in:-

Figure 18.1 Pi - Xin Relationship

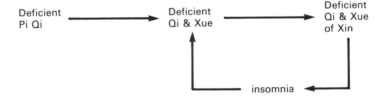

Thirdly, the relationship between Gan and Xin may have been impaired by the chronic depression, frustration, irritation and anger involved in his business stresses. This resulted in Depression of Gan Qi and Depression of Zong Qi, both leading to Stagnation of Qi and Xue in the chest region especially, and, in particular, to Stagnant Xin Xue.

In summary, the pattern of Stagnant Xin Xue is accompanied here by Deficient Xin Yang, Deficient Xin Qi, and Deficient Xin Xue; by Deficiency of both Shen and Pi; and by Depression of Gan Qi.

Treatment

Between attacks, combinations of points were selected from such as the following, and used with even method:-

Gongsun	SP.4	Confluent points of Chong Mai and Yin Wei Mai;
Neiguan	P.6	used to strengthen Shen, with moxa on Gongsun.
Juque	Ren 14	To strengthen Xin and Wei.
Shanzhong	Ren 17	To strengthen circulation of Zong Qi, to dispel stagnation, to regulate and to supress rebellious Qi, and expand the chest. Both Juque and Shanzhong used with moxa.
Shenshu	BL.23	To strengthen Qi and Yang of Shen.
Pishu	BL.20	To strengthen function of Pi to form Qi and Xue.
Geshu	BL.17	To strengthen circulation of Qi and Xue and to relieve Stagnation.
Xinshu	BL.15	To strengthen Qi and Yang of Xin. (All back Shu points used with moxa.)
Taichong	LIV.3	To relieve Depression of Gan Qi and Stagnation of Qi and Xue.

Patient Education
Great caution was advised with respect to physical exertion and exposure to Cold. The most difficult aspect was the combination of the deeply ingrained pattern of emotional disharmony with the excessive overwork. The patient was a perfectionist, and was advised to moderate this tendency, since it led to both permanent dissatisfaction with himself and others, and to an increased workload. He was advised to avoid emotional confrontations and conflicts of all natures wherever possible, since these would provide acute aggravation of Stagnation of Xin Xue, and possibly lead to another spell of continuous pain, or even to a full scale 'heart attack'. Various moderate activities of a relaxing, creative and social nature were suggested, to provide a break from the continual pattern of frustration and worry.

4.   Chest Pain

A man of 50 had chest pains at the age of 30, and on about 10 subsequent occasions. The last occurrence was in the January of the year he came for treatment, following working in the snow. On one occasion the pain was severe, but was generally dull, and of variable position, anywhere in the chest region, apparently in the muscles. It occurred any time, not necessarily immediately after physical work, and indeed, occasionally, when the patient was sitting down and relaxed, and not when he was active. There was catarrh and shortness of breath, and the last two fingers of both hands had numbness and tingling. Eighteen months ago he had had a sudden severe pain from the top of the spine to the head. From January onwards he had considerable anxiety, and there was much belching, but no other signs of digestive disharmony. The patient was overweight, somewhat sluggish, with cold feet; slippery but weak pulse; and pale flabby tongue with greasy coat.

Diagnosis
First of all, there are signs of Deficient Qi and Deficient Yang:- sluggishness, overweight, cold feet, weak pulse and pale flabby tongue. The catarrh, slippery yet empty pulse; and pale greasy tongue suggest Deficient Qi and Yang of Pi, resulting in formation of Phlegm.

Secondly, there were signs that at first sight might suggest Xin disharmony, specifically Deficient Xin Yang and Stagnant Xin Xue:- the chest pains, shortness of breath, and numbness and tingling going down into the last two fingers. Also, the chest pains were aggravated by Cold and exertion, for example working in the snow. However, this patient did not have a Xin disharmony. He did not have palpitations, the characteristic sign of Xin disharmony, nor the irregular pulse quality with which they are often associated. The shortness of breath was due to smoking cigarettes, not to Xin weakness, and the finger numbness derived from the trauma of the neck vertebrae. If it were Stagnant Xin Xue, the pain would be severe and stabbing, rather than dull; and a fixed rather than variable location. If Deficient Xin Yang were involved, the pain would be worse after exercise and improved on resting. In this case, on some occasions, the reverse was true.

From January, there had been considerable stress, and this was when both chest pain and belching began. In TCM, belching is usually due to Invasion of Pi by Gan Qi, following emotional stress or depression. This patient had a history of periodic ache in the chest and rib muscles. This may be due partly to inherent weakness in this area, and partly due to a sudden, unaccustomed use of the chest muscles, combined with Invasion by External Cold, as when working in the snow. Also, the general Deficiency of Qi and Yang tended to general poor circulation of Qi and Xue. This was aggravated by Depression of Gan Qi, due to stress, resulting in obstruction and irregular flow of Qi, and also Phlegm rising up to the chest and obstructing the channels and collaterals of the rib cage.

There was not a major Invasion of Cold, or the patient would have complained of coldness in the chest. Nor was there a major Depression of Gan Qi, or there would have been other Gan signs. Similarly, there was not a severe obstruction by Phlegm, or the patient would have complained of stuffiness and heaviness in the chest, rather than ache. Nor had the sudden use of the chest resulted in much injury to the chest muscles, since rather than aggravating the pain, further exercise tended to relieve it, suggesting Stagnation of Qi, relieved by movement. None of these factors was severe, but all combined together to produce the chest pain. The fact that pain was of variable rather than of fixed location, and was dull rather than severe, suggested Stagnation of Qi rather than Stagnation of Xue.

In summary, the local Deficiency and Stagnation of Qi in the muscles of the rib cage, with the dull pain of variable location, was associated with the combination of the following factors:-

General Deficient Qi and Deficient Yang
Phlegm resulting from Deficient Pi Qi and Deficient Pi Yang
Stagnation of Qi from:- sudden over-exertion of chest muscles
                    - pattern of previous weakness
                    - Depression of Gan Qi
                    - temporary Invasion by External Cold

Treatment

The following points were used with reinforcing method and moxa:-

Guanyuan	Ren 4	Strengthens Qi and Yang.
Qihai	Ren 6	Strengthens circulation of Qi.

Zhongwan	Ren 12	Strengthens Pi and Wei to eliminate Damp and Phlegm.
Shanzhong	Ren 17	Dispels Phlegm and fullness from the chest by invigorating circulation of Qi.
Neiguan	P.6	Regulates digestive system, opens the chest, and calms the mind.
Taichong	LIV.3	Regulates Gan to reduce Invasion of Pi by Gan, and removes Stagnation of Qi in the muscles of the chest region; calms the mind.

The chest pains had gone completely after four treatments, so treatment then concentrated on the numbness in the fingers, with occasional pain at the back of the neck:-

Houxi	SI.3 ⎱	The confluent points of the Du and Yang Qiao
Shenmai	BL.62 ⎰	channels, used to remove obstruction from Du Mai and to relax tendons and muscles. Also, Houxi is the local point for finger problems.
Dazhui	Du 14	Clears obstruction from Du channels, especially in the neck region.

These points were used with reinforcing method and moxa, and the finger problem was much better after two treatments.

Patient Education
The patient was advised to stop smoking, lose weight, and take regular gentle exercise; all of which he did, with good results. However, he become over-enthusiastic about the weight loss, became too thin, and started to lose strength. This mistake was corrected, and this patient remained well with treatment every 3 or 4 months.

5.   Urticaria and Stomach Pain

A Chinese woman of 34 came for treatment in Nanjing, having had stomach ache for 5 days and urticaria for 4 days. The urticaria was aggravated by wind. She had had intermittent stomach ache since childhood, and gastroptosis for 10 years. Her whole body was sensitive to cold, and during the stomach pain she liked warmth and pressure, warm foods such as chicken soup, and 'hot' foods such as ginger. She had loose stools, was easily affected by stress, her pulse was wiry and thin, and her tongue had a white coat.

Diagnosis
She had a chronic weakness of the Middle Jiao, i.e. a chronic Deficiency of Qi and Yang of both Pi and Wei, as shown by loose stools, thin pulse, and white tongue coat. This was associated with a general chronic Deficiency of Qi that enabled easy invasion of the Body by External Cold. Also, the weaker the Qi, the weaker the ability of the Qi to hold up the organs, and so the worse the stomach prolapse.

240

When the stomach was invaded by Cold, it would contract, producing a stabbing pain. Warmth, and warm and 'hot' food and drink, tended to dispel the Cold, and so gave relief. Pressure gave relief since the condition was one of Emptiness.

In Five Phase Theory, when Earth (Pi and Wei) is weak, the balance between Wood and Earth is upset, and Wood (Gan and Dan) may become hyperactive. This patient was prone to uprising Gan Qi, as shown by her wiry pulse and her reaction to stress. In this patient, three factors contributed to Heat in Xue; Gan hyperactivity, consumption of 'hot' foods, such as chicken and ginger; and exposure to External Wind.

In summary, External Cold had aggravated her chronic pattern of Internal Cold in the Middle Jiao, resulting in stomach pain; and the warming chicken soup and ginger, which relieved her stomach ache, had contributed to the urticaria. Gan hyperactivity, associated with stress, and exposure to External Wind, also contributed to the pattern of Heat in Xue, with which the urticaria was associated.

Treatment

The principle of treatment was to attend to the stomach ache and the urticaria at the same time; the former by strengthening and warming the Middle Jiao to dispel Cold and relieve pain; and the latter by dispelling Wind and Heat in Xue.

For the first treatment, the following points were used:-

Zhongwan	Ren 12	With moxa, to strengthen and warm Middle Jiao, dispel Cold and relieve pain.
Qihai	Ren 6	Strengthens Qi of whole Body to dispel Cold.
Zusanli	ST. 36	Strengthens Pi and Wei.
Quchi	LI. 11	
Sanjinjiao	SP. 6	Eliminate Heat in Xue.
Xuchai	SP. 10	

The very long needle treatment for stomach prolapse was not given to this patient. This method is useful for patients with a strong constitution, but this patient was too weak. She had had this treatment on a previous occasion, and improvement was neither complete nor lasting. Bahui, Du 20, may also be used with moxa for stomach prolapse, but was not used in this case since it would have aggravated the hyperactive Gan Qi.

Moxa may be used on Zhongwan, since this point warms Pi which tends to Cold and Damp, but should not be used in this patient on Quchi, Sanyinjiao and Xuehai. These points are used to remove Heat from Xue; moxa on them would increase the Heat in Xue, and aggravate the urticaria.

In this patient, some points were used to warm, simultaneously with other points which were used to cool.

The first treatment emphasized relief from pain and urticaria. Later treatments might add points such as Pishu, BL.20, to strengthen the constitution; and add points such as Fengmen, BL.12, and Fengchi, GB.20, to dispel Wind. Ganshu, BL.18, or Taichong, LIV.3, might be added to calm Gan, and Geshu, BL.17, to regulate Xue.

After six treatments, the patient felt less tired, and better than she had felt for a long time. Her urticaria was gone, although it tended to return slightly on exposure to Wind; and her stomach pain was greatly relieved, although still aggravated by Cold.

Patient Education

This patient was advised to avoid heavy work and lifting whenever possible, to avoid exposure to External Cold and to External Wind, to take warm nourishing food but not so much of the 'hot' type, and to avoid emotional stress whenever she could.

6.   Back, Shoulder, Breasts and Respiratory System

A woman of 43 had periodic lumbar soreness since a fall at 12 years, and for 2 years had had a severe pain radiating from shoulder to arm on the left side. For many years she had irritability, fluid retention, and lumpiness, distension and soreness of the breasts prior to menstruation. She had a tendency to occasional bursts of coughing and infection of the respiratory system. Her job was very demanding and stressful, and she had much worry and obsessive thinking about her work. She had had a severe uterine prolapse some years before, felt permanently tired, and was pale and overweight; with weak but wiry pulse; and pale purplish tongue.

Diagnosis

The area of potential weakness of circulation of Qi and Xue in the lower back was activated by the chronic condition of Deficient Qi and Deficient Yang. These Deficiencies were indicated by the pale face and tongue, tiredness, overweight, and empty pulse. The shoulder and arm problem, due to a sprain, was slow to heal due to low levels of Ying and Wei Qi. The constant overwork and worry led to weakness of Pi Qi, with consequent general Qi Deficiency and aggravation of weakness of Fei, since Fei depends on Pi for nourishment. Poor Transformation and Transportation by Pi of Jin Ye resulted in the fluid retention; and Deficient Pi Yang and subsequent inability of Pi to hold up organs, resulted in the uterine prolapse.

The premenstrual irritability and breast problem were due to Hyperactive Gan Yang, resulting from emotional stress and indicated by wiry pulse, affecting the Gan channel which passes through the breasts. Depression of Gan Qi and Hyperactive Gan Yang, indicated by purplish tongue, affected Pi, especially at period time, resulting in fluid retention. Weakness of Wei Qi in general, and Fei Qi in particular, led to a tendency to Invasion of Fei by External Disease Factors, resulting in patterns of Heat in Fei - as in viral pneumonia, or coughing, due to impaired Dispersing function of Fei.

Treatment

Treatment was in four areas:-

    Back and General
    Shoulder and General
    Breast and Fluid Retention
    Respiratory Problems

Back and General
The following points were used with even method:-

Sanyinjiao	SP.6	Strengthens Pi and Shen and regulates Gan.
Pishu	BL.20	Strengthens Pi to produce Qi and Xue.
Shenshu	BL.23	Strengthens Shen and back.
Dachangshu	BL.25	Strengthens and invigorates channels of the lower back.

There was a great improvement after this single treatment, both in lumbar ache and in general feeling of health. After one more such treatment, the third treatment was on the shoulders.

Shoulder and General
The following points were used with even method, and the points specifically for shoulder and neck were used on the left side only:-

Sanyinjiao	SP.6	Regulates Pi, Shen and Gan.
Taichong	LIV.3	Regulates Gan to dispel Stagnation and pacify Yang.
Binao	LI.14	Invigorate circulation of Qi and Xue in the channels and collaterals of shoulder and arm.
Jugu	LI.16	
Tianliao	TB.15	
Chonggu	M-HN-31	Invigorate circulation of Qi and Xue in the channels and collaterals of neck and shoulder.
Qijingzhuipang	N-BW-3	

Breasts and Fluid Retention
When fluid retention was a problem, the following points were used with even method, and with moxa on the first two points only:-

Qihai	Ren 6	Invigorates Qi circulation to dispel Damp.
Shuifen	Ren 9	Specific point for fluid retention on Ren channel.
Sanyinjiao	SP.6	Strengthen Pi to dispel Damp
Yinlingquan	SP.9	
Taichong	LIV.3	Reduces Invasion of Pi by Gan, and hence strengthens Pi to dispel Damp.

When dealing with lumpiness, distension and soreness of the breasts, the following points were selected and used with even method. If distension and soreness were considerable, reducing method was used, and if soreness was severe, Taichong and Qimen were joined on the right side with electro- acupuncture.

Taichong	LIV.3	Pacify Hyperactive Gan Yang, disperse obstruction of circulation of Qi and Xue in the breasts.
Qimen	LIV.14	
Rugen	ST.18	Regulates Qi in the breasts, since Wei channel passes through them.

Respiratory Problems

When respiratory problems occurred, such points as the following were used with even method, exept Kongzhui, which was used with reducing method in acute situations.

Kongzhui	LU.6	Eliminates Heat, regulates Fei Qi, helps Fei Qi descend; especially for acute disorders.
Taiyuan	LU.9	Strengthens Fei, stops coughing.
Susanli	ST.36	Strengthens Pi and Wei to produce Ying Qi and Wei Qi, to nourish and protect Fei.
Feishu	BL.13	Eliminates Wind and Heat from Fei, regulates circulation of Fei Qi, and especially the dispersing function.
Dazhui	Du 14	Eliminates External Factors, for example Wind Cold and Heat.

Patient Education

The main advice to this patient was to get more rest, and to find more pleasant social activity and relaxation away from the pressures and worries of the job. This was difficult at the time of treatment, since she was in the middle of selling her house, and in an especially demanding phase of the job. She was recommended not to take on any further workload, and to plan a reduction of work in the future. Also, when she had moved house she was advised not to plan any great alterations and renovations, until she had recovered her strength. Also, since in TCM, Gan is responsible for planning and Dan for decisions and judgments, it is best to avoid making major plans and decisions when the mind is tired and when under mental and emotional distress.

7.   Debility and Insomnia

A man of 32 had lack of energy and a tendency to cold feet, and yet feelings of heat in the upper Body and especially the head. He suffered from insomnia, restlessness and irritability; with occasional headaches, lower back pain and depression. He had periodic indigestion, and his stools were loose, occasionally with particles of undigested food. His pulse was slippery and wiry yet empty, and occasionally fast. His tongue was pale and flabby, red at the edges and tip, and with a greasy coat that was sometimes white and sometimes yellowish.

Diagnosis

This is a case of chronic Internal Deficiency, showing some signs of Deficient Heat and Deficient Yin, and some signs of Deficient Cold and Deficient Yang. This case illustrates the principles discussed on page 22, since here is a pattern of overall Deficiency of Qi, in which sometimes Deficient Yin predominates, and at other times Deficient Yang predominates; and in which some Zang Fu are in a state of Deficient Yin, whilst at the same time others are tending to Deficient Yang.

General Deficient Qi is indicated by the lack of energy, pale flabby tongue and empty pulse. Deficiency of Shen Qi is indicated by the lumbar soreness, Deficient

Shen Yang by the cold extremities, and Deficient Pi Qi and Yang by the loose stools with occasional particles of undigested food. These signs of Deficient Yang and Qi of Shen and Pi were generally aggravated by Cold and tiredness from overwork.

The feelings of Heat in the upper Body, restlessness, insomnia, irritability, occasional rapid pulse, and tongue with some areas of redness, indicate Deficient Yin. The lumbar soreness indicates Deficient Yin of Shen, the red sides of the tongue Deficient Yin of Gan, and the red tip of the tongue Deficient Yin of Xin. The headaches and wiry pulse indicate Invasion of Gan, the depression suggests Depression of Gan Qi; and the periodic indigestion, empty slippery pulse and greasy tongue, indicate Invasion of Pi by Gan. The signs of Heat and Deficient Yin were generally aggravated by mental overwork and stress and by emotional disturbance.

Treatment
The treatment of this patient depended on whether the Deficient Yin or the Deficient Yang was temporarily predominant. If the weather was cold and the patient tired, it was possible to strengthen the Deficient Yang, and even to use moxa, providing the pulse was not fast, there were no signs of Heat, and that the patient was going to have a quiet time in the days following treatment. If, however, the patient had been under mental and emotional stress, and was showing signs of Deficient Yin, the treatment would aim more at nourishing the Yin, in order to control the rising Yang and Fire of Gan and Xin.

Principal Points

Guanyuan	Ren 4	Strengthens Shen Qi.
Qihi	Ren 6	Strengthens Qi circulation.
Zhongwan	Ren 12	Strengthens Qi of Pi and Wei.
Zusanli	ST.36	Strengthens Pi and Wei and regulated circulation of Qi and Xue.
Shenshu	BL.23	Strengthens Shen Qi.
Pishu	BL.20	Strengthens Pi Qi.
Ganshu	BL.18	Removes Stagnation of Gan Qi.
Taichong	LIV.3	Removes Stagnation of Gan Qi and pacifies Hyperactive Gan Yang, to reduce Invasion of Pi by Gan, and to calm the mind.

Points were selected from this group, depending on the conditions, and were used with even method.

Deficient Yang Predominates
When Deficient Yang predominated, moxa was used, providing there were no signs of Heat, on Guanyuan, Qihi, Zhongwan, Zusanli, Shenshu and Pishu, and, in addition, Mingmen, Du 4. Again, even method of needling was used.

Deficient Yin Predominates
Needles were used with even method, but with no moxa, and, in addition to points selected from the principal group, or as alternatives to them, the following points were used:-

Xingjian	LIV.2	To pacify rising Gan Yang and Fire.
Sanyinjiao	SP.6	To strengthen Yin of Shen, Pi and Gan.
Taixi	KID.3	To nourish Yin.
Tongli	HE.5	To calm mind and Xin. To bring down fire from head caused by mental irritation.

The basic problem with such a patient, in any given treatment, is deciding whether to build him up or calm him down. This depends on the condition and situation of the patient at a particular treatment. For example, one treatment of this patient was given after a prolonged bout of mental over-exertion and emotional stress, with general rushing about:-

Baihui	Du 20	To calm mind by calming disordered Yang and Qi in the Head.
Yintang	M-HN-3	To clear and calm mind.
Taichong	LIV.3	To regulate Gan and calm the mind.
Yongquan	KID.1	To nourish Yin, calm Fire of Gan and Xin, and calm the mind.

Even method was used, and the patient felt drowsy and relaxed after the treatment, which was given in the evening. It would be pointless to give such a treatment to such a patient during the day, since he would simply rush off immediately afterwards at his usual hectic pace, and spoil the treatment. In this particular case, telling the patient not to rush around after the treatment would have little effect, since the habit was so deeply ingrained.

Patient Education
Appropriate action for the patient in this case would first and foremost be to slow down the rushed and hectic pace, and to plan periods of rest and relaxation, in order to restore the Deficiencies of Qi, Yang and Yin. However, this patient's lifestyle had become so habitual and the patient's drive to overwork was so great, that change in this area was both small and slow. Somewhat better progress was made in regularizing eating habits and in avoiding excess rich food and alcohol, so as to reduce the Invasion of Pi by Gan. However, overall, this case is an example of more help being given by acupuncture than by patient education. It is possible that, in time, and especially if the patient really overloads himself and suffers a 'nervous breakdown', the motivation for personal change may increase.

8.   Arthritis and Stress

A woman of 70 had pain in the joints of the hands, shoulders, neck, lower spine, hips and knees. This pain was of fixed location, aggravated by cold and alleviated by warmth. She also had indigestion, nausea, bitter taste, and periodic pain in the epigastric and in the right hypochondriac region. She suffered from irritability, hypersensitivity, headache, dizziness, insomnia and periodic eczema. These symptoms were aggravated by emotional stress which was continual with periodic severe crises. She had a dull pale face, pale lips, felt weakness and lack of energy, and had the early stages of cataracts. Her pulse was empty thin choppy and wiry; and her tongue was pale and flabby.

Diagnosis

This case, with its complexity, chronic Deficiency and stress, is typical of many in the West. In fact, the case was considerably more complex than outlined here, where only the essentials are dealt with for the sake of simplicity.

The pattern was one of chronic Internal Deficiency, with periodic exacerbations due to stress; and both Zang Fu and Jing Luo were involved. The dull pale face, pale lips and tongue, thin choppy pulse, and weakness, suggest Deficient Xue. The dizziness and insomnia may be due to Deficient Xue, or to Deficient Yin and Hyperactive Yang. The lack of energy, emptiness of the pulse and flabby tongue, suggest Deficient Qi, in addition to Deficient Xue. Also, in TCM, optic degeneration may be due to insufficient Qi and Xue to nourish the eyes.

Deficient Yin and Hyperactive Yang of Gan resulted in the irritability, hypersensitivity, headache, dizziness, insomnia, and thin wiry pulse. Depression of Gan Qi was associated here with depression of emotion; depression of the flow of bile, hence the bitter taste and hypochondriac pain; and Invasion of Pi and Wei, leading to indigestion, nausea and epigastric pain. Chronic eczema, in TCM, may be due to Heat lodging in Xue, in cases of Deficient Xue, but here, the fact that the eczema only occurred in periods of severe emotional crisis, suggested that the Heat in Xue might also be associated patterns of Damp Heat in Gan and Dan, and Fire in Gan. Deficiency and imbalance of Gan would also tend to affect the eyes.

The pain in the joints, which was of fixed location, aggravated by Cold and alleviated by warmth, corresponds to the pattern of Fixed Bi in TCM. This patient had done much heavy manual labour in the past, with considerable wear and tear on the joints, producing foci of bone deterioration and weakness of circulation of Qi and Xue, which, with age and Deficiency of Qi and Xue, became worse, causing pain.

Treatment

There are four main areas for treatment:-

Deficient Qi and Xue
Gan Disharmonies
Fixed Bi
Eye Disorders

With this patient, there were too many disorders to treat them all in any one session; too many needles would be required, and this patient, due to weakness and stress, would be likely to faint. Therefore, it was necessary to produce a long-term plan of treatment. However, the results of emotional crisis had to be treated when they occurred, causing temporary departure from the planned treatment schedule.

Deficient Qi and Xue

Points were selected from such as the following, and used with reinforcing method. Caution was needed with the use of moxa, especially on points connecting with the Yin organs, since this patient tended to Yin Deficiency, especially in times of emotional crisis.

Qihai	Ren 6	To strengthen Qi and circulation of Qi.
Zusanli	ST.36	To strengthen Qi and Xue, and their circulation.
Xuehai	SP.10	Regulates circulation of Ying Qi and Xue. Also clears Heat from Xue, as in eczema.
Sanyinjiao	SP.6	Strengthens function of Pi and Wei to form Qi and Xue, strengthens circulation of Qi and Xue. Clears Heat from Xue, as in eczema.
Gongsun	SP.4	Strengthens Pi, Wei and Chong Mai. Relieves pain, especially in epigastric region.
Pishu	BL.20	Strengthens Pi and Xue.
Geshu	BL.17	Invigorates circulation of Xue.
Xinshu	BL.15	Invigorates circulation of Qi and Xue.

Gan Disharmonies

Points, such as the following, would be used with even method:-

Taichong	LIV.3	Regulates Gan to relieve Depression of Qi and pacify Hyperactive Yang.
Yanglingquan	GB.34	Relieves Damp Heat in Gan and Dan, Pacifies Hyperactive Yang.
Fengchi	GB.20	Pacifies Yang and clears the mind; to strengthen the eyes.
Baihui	Du 20	To pacify Yang and calm the mind.
Yintang	M-HN-3	To clear and calm the mind, to relieve tension and headache, dizziness and insomnia.

Fixed Bi

Points, such as those below, were used with reinforcing method and with moxa:-

Hands	Sanjian, LI.3; Hegu, LI.4; Yangxi, LI.5.
Shoulders	Binao, LI.14; Jianyu, LI.15; Jugu, LI.16; Jianneiling, M-UE-48.
Neck	Dazhui, Du 14; Chuanhsi (Special Point).
Lower Spine	Yaoyangguan, Du 3; Guanyuanshu, BL.26; Baliao, BL.31-34; Shiqizhuixia, N-BW-25.
Hips	Huantiao, GB.30; Yanglingquan, GB.34; Juegu, GB.39.
Knees	Xiyan, ST.35; Xixia, M-LE-15; Heding, M-LE-27; In addition to Zusanli, Xuehai, Yinglingquan and Yanglingquan.

Eye Disorders

For the initial stages of cataract, and the generally weak vision, points from the following list would be used with gentle insertion and minimal manipulation. In addition to Taichong, Yanlingquan, Yintang and Fengchi; the following points might be added:-

Guangming, GB.37; Tongziliao, GB.1; Zanzhu, BL.2 (through to Jingming); Jingming, BL.1; Chengqi, ST.1; Yiming, M-HN-13; Qiuhou, M-HN-8; Touguangming, M-HN-5; Yuyao, M-HN-6.

Patient Education

This patient needed rest, relaxation and quiet, and specifically needed to avoid heavy work, lifting, or exposure to Cold, that would tend to aggravate the pain in the joints. The main source of stress for this individual was the very great difficulty suffered with and by members of her family, and there was very little that the patient or the practitioner could do to reduce her worry and anxiety in this area. She was advised to avoid arguments or situations of emotional stress, as far as it was possible to do so. She was encouraged to take up her old pastimes of painting and gardening, since gentle pottering at these activities took her mind off her worries and allowed her to relax.

In this case, nutrition was most important. Firstly, to support the Deficiency of Qi and Xue, an adequate, balanced diet was organised. Secondly, iron supplement was given to support the Deficient Xue, and complete B vitamin complex was given to counteract the effects of tiredness and stress on the nervous system. Thirdly, since there was hypersensitivity of both Gan and Wei to fatty, sugary or spicy foods, and to strong tea or coffee and alcohol, these had to be greatly reduced. This patient was concerned about being overweight, and periodically starved herself in an attempt to reduce it. Since this practice tended to aggravate the Deficiency or both Pi and Wei, the patient was persuaded to avoid it.

Although emotional crisis produced temporary attacks, the combination of treatment and patient education was gradually effective in this case, in all four areas, but mainly in arresting the deterioration, rather than restoration to perfect health. Also, the effects of all but the most severe crises could be ameliorated to some degree.

Summary of Case Histories

In TCM, it can be seen from the eight case histories above that:-

1. The entire process of diagnosis, treatment and patient education is in terms of:- Eight Principles, Disease Factors, Substances, Jing Luo and Zang Fu. This is the framework on which all clinical practice is based.

2. In each of the eight cases, even the simpler ones, there were at least six patterns of disharmony of Zang Fu and Jing Luo involved in each. This emphasises the need for the practitioner to be thoroughly fluent with general theory, clinical theory, and clinical technique, if there is to be any hope of accurate diagnosis, of disentangling the various threads of apparently conflicting evidence, and of weaving a clear pattern.

3. Besides the various patterns of disharmony involved in the major illness, there may be one or more subsidiary disharmonies, some of which may have little connection to the main disorder. For example, in case history 6, there are four separate patterns of disharmony, two of which are mainly Jing Luo patterns, and two of which are predominantly Zang Fu patterns. Although all four are linked by the general condition of Deficiency of Qi, they arose as four separate areas of illness. This is very common in the West, where an individual patient may present with a whole range of chronic disorders.

Chapter
19

Conclusion

Review

Part 1 surveyed the background to the Theory of Zang Fu.
Chapter 1 considered the essential differences between Chinese and Western thought, and the great dangers of applying Western thinking, Western concepts and Western medical terminology to Chinese medicine.

Chapter 2 discussed the organisational framework of the Body:- the Substances, Jing Luo, Zang Fu, and Tissues. Chapter 3 studied the Substances in detail, since an understanding of their functions, origins and Patterns of Disharmony, is essential to an understanding of Zang Fu. Chapters 4 and 5 discussed the origins and patterns of disease.

Part 2 was concerned with the individual Zang Fu.
Chapter 6 briefly looked at the origins of confusion regarding Western study of Zang Fu; and Chapters 7 to 11 discussed the functions, Origins of Disease and Patterns of Disharmony of the Five Zang and their paired Fu. General guidelines for choice of points were given for each Pattern of Disharmony.

Chapter 12 briefly considered Xin Bao, then examined various facets of the San Jiao concept. Chapter 13 reviewed the Zang Fu by observing how each Pattern of Disharmony originates from failure of a particular Zang function.

Part 3 dealt with Zang Fu interrelationships.
Chapter 14 viewed Zang Fu interrelationships in the context of Yin Yang, Substances, Jing Luo, and Tissues; and examined the types of interrelationships between Zang Fu, and between Zang Fu and the Origins of Disease.

Chapter 15 looked at Zang Fu interrelationships in terms of the emotions, and considered the clinical importance, and the treatment, of various emotional disharmonies.

Chapter 16 investigated the Patterns of Disharmony of eleven Zang pairs; then considered disharmonies of three or more Zang together, especially in the areas of emotional disharmony, digestive problems, and gynaecological and obstetric disorders; and finally looked at Zang Fu interrelationships in some Common Disease Patterns.

Part 4 examined the application of Zang Fu theory in clinical practice.
Chapter 17 briefly dealt with diagnosis, treatment and the education of the patient; and gave a simple sequence of clinical procedures.

Chapter 18 studied eight case histories of increasing complexity, which illustrated the application of Zang Fu theory in clinical practice with actual patients.

General

Chinese thought is not Western thought, and the Zang Fu are not the organs of Western medicine. This book has discussed the functions, Origins of Disharmony, and Patterns of Disharmony of Zang Fu, in the context of TCM as a whole, and in terms of interrelationships. This presents a very different picture from the physiology, pathology and syndromes of the organs of Western medicine.

The concept of interrelationship is absolutely fundamental to the theory and practice of Chinese medicine, and is a recurring theme throughout this book. All the manifestations of the Zang Fu, in health and in disease, are based on patterns of interrelationship that change and develop throughout the life of the individual.

The emphasis throughout has been on clinical practice; theory has not been described for its own sake. Furthermore, although many practical examples have been given in the text, the only way that TCM can be learned is by many years experience of applying the theoretical principles in the clinic. Only in this way is it possible to learn to differentiate the many possible permutations and combinations of disharmonies that occur in clinical practice. However, we do not deal with combinations of disharmonies, we deal with people, and the understanding in depth of the emotional, mental and spiritual needs of people, lies outside the scope of this book.

Teaching TCM

The aim of any course teaching TCM is to provide students with a clear framework of theoretical understanding, and with the skills and techniques to apply these theoretical principles in clinical practice.

This involves an understanding of the principles of Chinese thought and Chinese philosophy, without which there can be no true comprehension of TCM.

The Basic Theoretical Framework
The basic theoretical framework has been discussed, and comprises a thorough understanding of the interrelationships between the following six categories:-

Yin Yang	Substances
Eight Principles	Jing Luo
Disease Factors	Zang Fu

There are other facets of TCM which should be studied, such as the Six Divisions, the Classification of Warm Diseases, and the Theory of the Five Phases; but compared to the basic framework of the above six categories, these are of relatively minor importance in the clinical practice of acupuncture.

This basic theoretical framework is the central part of the courses run by the colleges of Beijing, Guangzhou, Nanjing, and Shanghai, in the People's Republic of China. Eventually, it will become the common core of the curricula of the Western Colleges. Each Western college may specialise in one or more aspects of TCM, such as Eight Extra Channels, Stems and Branches, or Five Phase Theory, but it is essential that they share this basic common core.

Traditional and Chinese
In teaching TCM, it is most important that the basic theoretical framework is both Traditional and Chinese. If material from other countries and other cultures is mixed in with the basic TCM framework, then the student cannot fully understand TCM, and misconceptions will occur, reducing clinical efficiency.

It is always best to learn one system at a time, and to understand it fully before moving on to another. In the case of TCM, it takes much time to assimilate and to practise properly, and the students must exert the patience and self-discipline to do this, before attempting to blend TCM with other systems. For example, the Japanese, Korean and Vietnamese systems each have great value in themselves, but it is unwise to mix material from these systems in with TCM in the early years of training. It is vital that students learn to diagnose, differentiate and treat, in terms of TCM alone, so that they fully understand the theoretical principles and master the practical techniques, before extending to other systems.

Ambiguity
There are many areas of difficulty and ambiguity for the Western student in learning TCM. It is most important in teaching Chinese medicine that these areas are neither avoided on the one hand, nor given hard-and-fast, clear-cut resolutions on the other. Flexibility and ambiguity are two of the greatest strengths of Chinese medicine, since medicine deals with people, and people themselves are complex, fluid, ambiguous, and always changing and developing.

Theory and Practice
It is vitally important in teaching TCM, that there is not a great separation between the teaching of theory and the teaching of practice. Theory and practice are mutually dependent, and ideally part of each day should be devoted to practice and part to theory; part of the day spent in the lecture room, and part in the clinic. Theoretical understanding increases clinical ability, and clinical experience strengthens and develops theoretical understanding. Theoretical principles only have life and relevance when they are manifested in practice. It is one thing to learn about a phenomenon in theory, and it is a very different thing to experience it in life. There is a great gulf between merely knowing something intellectually, and having that knowledge embodied by experience. The concern of TCM is not merely with theory, but with experience and with people.

252

Appendix

List of Zang Functions and Disharmonies

Zang	Functions	Patterns of Disharmony
Shen	Stores Jing:- Rules reproduction & growth Rules Bones Foundation of Yin Yang Rules Water Rules Reception of Qi Opens into Ears; Manifests in Hair	Deficient Shen Jing Deficient Shen Yang Shen Qi Not Firm Shen Fails to Receive Qi Water Overflowing Deficient Shen Yin
Pi	Rules Transformation & Transportation Rules Muscles & Limbs Governs Xue Holds up Organs Opens into Mouth; Manifests in Lips	Deficient Pi Qi Deficient Pi Yang Inability of Pi to Govern Xue Sinking of Pi Qi Invasion of Pi by Cold & Damp Damp Heat Accumulates in Pi
Gan	Rules Free-flowing of Qi Stores Xue Rules Tendons Opens into Eyes; Manifests in Nails	Depression of Gan Qi Deficient Gan Xue Hyperactive Gan Yang Blazing Gan Fire Stirring of Gan Wind Damp Heat in Gan & Dan Stagnation of Cold in Gan Jing Luo
Xin	Rules Xue & Xue Mai Stores Shen* Opens into Tongue; Manifests in Face	Deficient Xin Qi Deficient Xin Yang Collapse of Xin Yang Stagnant Xin Xue Deficient Xin Xue Deficient Xin Yin Blazing Xin Fire Phlegm Fire Agitating Xin Cold Phlegm Misting Xin
Fei	Rules Qi & Governs Respiration Governs Dispersing & Descending Regulates Water Channels Rules Exterior of Body Opens into Nose; Manifests in Body Hair	Deficient Fei Qi Deficient Fei Yin Invasion of Fei by Wind Retention of Phlegm in Fei
Xin Bao	Protects Xin Guides Joy & Pleasure	Heat Affecting Xin Bao Phlegm Obstructing Xin Bao

List of Fu Functions and Disharmonies

Fu	Functions	Patterns of Disharmony
Pang Guang	Receives & Excretes Urine	Damp Heat in Pang Guang (various types) Deficient Pang Guang Qi (see Deficient Shen Yang)
Wei	Receiving & Ripening of Food & Drink	Retention of Fluid in Wei due to Cold Retention of Food in Wei Deficient Wei Yin Blazing Wei Fire Stagnant Xue in Wei
Dan	Stores & Secretes Bile	(see Damp Heat in Gan & Dan) Deficient Dan Qi
Xiao Chang	Separates Pure from Impure	Obstructed Qi of Xiao Chang Excess Heat in Xiao Chang Deficient Cold in Xiao Chang (see Deficient Pi Qi) Stagnant Qi odf Xiao Chang (see Stagnation of Cold in Gan Jing Luo)
Da Chang	Receives Impure and Eliminates Faeces	Intestinal Abcess Exhausted Fluid of Da Chang Damp Heat Invades Da Chang Cold Damp in Da Chang (see Invasion of Pi by Cold & Damp) Deficient Da Chang Qi (see Deficient Pi Yang)
San Jiao	Regulates Jin Ye Metabolism	Does not have disharmonies separable from the disharmonies of other Zang Fu

Bibliography

1 'Acupuncture Charts', (China Cultural Corporation), 1975
2 'Heal Thyself', Bach E., (C.W.Daniel), 1974
3 Chen Qing Hua, London Seminar, 1984
4 'The Tao of Physics', Capra F., (Fontana), 1976
5 'Differential Diagnosis and Treatment of TCM', Cheung C.S. & Yat-Ki Lai, (TCM Publishers), 1980
6 Course Notes, Beijing College of TCM
7 Course Notes, Nanjing College of TCM, 1982
8 Course Notes, Zhongsan Medical College, Guangzhou, 1981
9 'Essentials of Chinese Acupuncture', (Foreign Languages Press Beijing), 1980
10 'An Explanatory Book of the Newest Illustrations of Acupuncture Points' (Medicine and Health Publishing Co.), 1978
11 'I Ching', trans. R. Wilhelm, (Routledge & Kegan Paul), 1974
12 'The Web That Has No Weaver', Kaptchuk T.J., (Congdon & Weed), 1983
13 'Current Acupuncture Therapy', Lee J.F. & Cheung C.S., (Medical Book Publications), 1978
14 'Pulse Diagnosis', Li Shi Zhen, (Transl. Hoc Hu Huynh), 1981
15 Li Zhe Ming & Ye Cheng Ku, Journal of Chinese Medicine No. 9, 1982
16 'Chinese Medical Terminology', Liu F. & Liu Yan Mau, (Commercial Press) 1980
17 'Tongue Diagnosis in Color', Lu H.C., (Academy of Oriental Heritage)
18 'Acupuncture - a Comprehensive Text', transl. O'Connor J. & Bensky D., (Eastland Press), 1981
19 'The Theoretical Foundations of Chinese Medicine', Porkert M., (M.I.T. Press), 1974
20 British Journal of Acupuncture, Vol. 6, No.1, Ross J., 1983

256

21 Journal of Chinese Medicine, No. 11, Ross J., 1983
22 Journal of Chinese Medicine, No. 12, Ross J., 1983
23 'Chinese Medicine', Shen J.H., (Educational Solutions), 1980
24 London Seminar of J.H. Shen, 1978
25 Personal Communication, Su Xin Ming
26 'The Bach Remedies Repertory', Wheeler F.J., (C.W. Daniel) 1974
27 'Chinese Pulse Diagnosis' We Shui Wan, 1973
28 Personal Communication, Wu Xinjin, 1981.

Index

INDEX

INDEX

INDEX